CONTENTS

SECTION TWO   Exercising

SECTION THREE Persevering

SOFT STEPS

It's as simple as this: Apply the steps in this book, and you'll reduce fat, reshape your muscles, and be a happier and more productive person for it.

This manual is divided into three sections—Eating, Exercising, and Persevering—and contains 98 soft steps. By soft steps, I mean small and easy-to-understand guides that you can apply to your lifestyle. Brought together and practiced consistently, they can transform your body into a leaner, stronger, healthier machine.

You are about to take charge of your life. You are going to eat better, exercise better, and live better.

A hard body can be yours—sooner than you think.

Get started today!

EATING

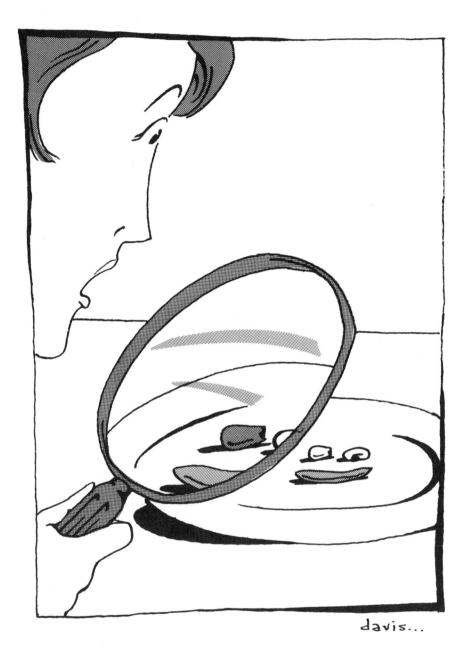

How small is small?

1

Eat Small Meals for Big Benefits

If you're looking for an almost pain-free way to shed several pounds, there may be a better strategy than cutting calories. Eating the same food but spreading the calories more evenly throughout the day might have a surprising impact.

Yes, the answer could be smaller and more frequent dosages of calories that by day's end total the same as you're now eating. This seeming phenomenon is based on an understanding of metabolism, which is the rate at which our bodies convert food into energy (which it burns) or fat (which it stores).

Metabolism is a sensitive mechanism that speeds up or slows down depending on the demand. Just like our highways handling traffic flow, there are only so many calories our bodies can process at one time.

When we starve ourselves—even if only for several hours—our metabolic rates slow. Think of an eight-lane freeway contracting into just two lanes, or even one. Then rush hour hits. Boom. Pouring calories onto a metabolic-rate slowdown means that more calories will be stored as fat.

Advice to eat more frequently stems from research done by Dr. Bryant Stamford, head of the Health Promotion and Wellness Center at the University of Louisville. In one study, 80 percent of the obese people surveyed were eating less than people of normal weight, but they were eating it all in one meal.

Dr. Stamford says one massive meal a day is the worst way to care for the body. The second worst way, he says, is only two meals per day. Big meals tend to produce big waistlines, Dr. Stamford contends.

There are at least three reasons why one-meal-a-day dieting is a poor method for shedding fat:

♦ It tends to turn into gorging.

♦ The body perceives starvation and thus slows the metabolic rate to compensate.

♦ The body cannot accommodate a large amount of food at once.

Large meals trigger extra amounts of insulin to break down the food. They also promote the conversion of carbohydrates, which include sugar, into fat.

A couple of hundred calories every three hours keeps us on an even keel—never stuffed and never famished. While convenience may be an issue, six eating episodes per day is advisable. An eating episode is a meal, snack, or nibble. While some episodes will likely result in more calories than others, try to match them as evenly as possible.

2

Three Easy Actions to Better Eating Habits

You're going to start your diet and exercise program Monday . . . or the day after. In the meantime, you'll have another glass of wine and some cheese and crackers.

You're always going to start tomorrow. But be honest with yourself: This is merely a game aimed at reducing guilt.

Begin to improve your eating habits now. Emphasize improvement. Don't expect to flip a switch and find perfection. For the next several weeks, try to incorporate the following habits into your eating patterns:

♦ **Eat your diet dessert first.**
   It takes sugar about twenty minutes to work its way through your system. By starting your meal with something sweet, you're more likely to feel satisfied at the end. Since most pies are 300 to 450 calories per piece (a piece is one-sixth of a pie), the calorie savings can be astronomical. Switch to a fat-free, frozen dessert, about 200 calories per slice.

♦ **Skim the fat from milk products.**
   One cup of whole milk contains 148 calories, almost half of them dietary fat. Milk with 2 percent fat (according to weight, not calories) contains 120 calories, of which 38 percent are fat. Skim milk has only a trace of fat in its 90 calories per cup.

   If your taste buds resist the change, gear down gradually. Go from whole milk to 2 percent to 1 percent to skim.

◆ **Fill up on fiber.**

The recommended daily fiber intake for adults is 35 to 50 grams per day. You'll get more fiber by emphasizing whole-wheat breads, whole-grain cereals, fruits, vegetables and legumes. Eating these foods tends to decrease consumption of foods high in fat. Broccoli is high in fiber and loaded with nutrients. Cup for cup, it has more fiber than cauliflower, spinach, cabbage, or string beans.

Keep plenty of fruits and vegetables around the house. It is easier to resist temptation if you're full, and these fiber-rich foods go a good deal further than pastries, cookies and chips.

Kidney beans are another good fiber source, containing three times more dietary fiber than green beans. Raspberries have four times the fiber of cherries.

See how many substitutions you can make. Identify the food you normally eat, then try to find a replacement that offers more fiber.

Don't try to change too much too quickly. Concentrate on developing these three habits. Soon it will seem natural to eat your fat-free dessert first, consume only skim-milk products and emphasize high-fiber foods.

You're not likely to knock off 20 pounds in a month. But if you make these three changes, one year from now you should be 10 pounds thinner, and your new habits should enable you to stay that way for a long time.

3

Don't Get Caught by Diet-Fad Traps

Perhaps you're one of those people who've never seen a diet gimmick you haven't fallen for. You notice someone looking a little thinner, and you find out how they did it. As more and more discover the secret, the buzz goes out through a legion of diet heads eager for the magical formula they think is going to transform their lives.

The current craze of the diet heads is a high-fiber diet cookie. Eating this cookie along with some water—to ignite its expansion in your stomach—provides abundant satiety, they say, meaning you're full enough to fend off further calorie consumption.

Three of these cookies with water each day and you'll indeed lose weight. You'll continue slimming down as long as it's a novelty, as long as this gimmick captures your imagination, and until you absolutely can't stand the taste or sight of the cookie any more. Without proper exercise, much of the weight you'll lose from this severe calorie deprivation will be lean muscle and organ tissue. There will be some fat-cell deflation, too, but only about half the weight shown on the scale will have come from flab. Without proper exercise, you'll still be the same shape, just a smaller version of it.

But the worst thing that happens is that your body's calorie-burning engine (metabolism) will decelerate to conserve its famine-fighting fat stores. Your body parts with fat only grudgingly.

The situation that develops is this:

◆ The over-dosage of the cookies, cakes, or whatever one-food magic formula you're using eventually makes them repulsive to you.

◆ The wasting away of needed lean tissue lowers your body's calorie-burning rate.

◆ You revert to your old eating habits and start storing fat like never before.

How many times do you have to go through this cycle before you realize it just leaves you fatter than you ever used to be?

The elements of a healthy, fit lifestyle are good eating and exercising habits day after day, month after month, year after year, decade after decade, and beyond.

Attempts to short-cut this proven method backfire.

The reason this cookie thing won't work is that it doesn't solve the problem. The Cambridge Diet, the Grapefruit Diet, the Hard-Boiled Egg Diet and the assortment of other gimmicks that have come down the pike have all provided short-term weight loss and long-term fatness.

The problem with being fat isn't that we're hungry, at least not physiologically hungry. A cookie that fills you up, or fasting program that keeps you from feeling hunger, is not in the ballpark of the basic problem.

The problem is that we like to eat. We enjoy the taste of food, both in our mouths and in our bellies. We are prompted to consume calories for a great many emotional and social reasons, regardless of whether or not we feel full.

Diet quackery is a thriving industry because so many of us want to side-step the real issue.

Learn about the basic food groups, the essential vitamins and minerals, and the triggers that set off our individual desires to eat. Don't think that after you lose all the weight you want using this diet cookie that you'll then become a student of good eating—you won't.

A quick, potent, filling bar or cookie still leaves my mouth wanting something to chomp on and my tastebuds something to salivate over. Quick calories aren't as useful as those you can really chew on.

Imagine a lean chicken breast, a red potato, some green beans and applesauce and maybe a small salad—now *there's* a symphony of tastebud delights.

Learn to eat a balanced diet, and stop eating when you're no longer hungry. Don't confuse eating until no longer hungry with eating until full. There are lots of calories between those two points, and slicing off the excess will probably result in a similar occurrence on your body.

If you have to tote along something convenient for long spells between meals, try a banana, whole wheat bread, matzo crackers, or a fig bar.

4

Pounds Lost on Liquid Diets Are Easy to Find

Quick weight loss is the appeal of most liquid diets featuring a ridiculously low number of calories, usually 400 to 800 per day.

These diets provide little more than temporary excitement. Your boomerang will come back.

Many dieters will regain their lost weight—on as few as 1000 calories per day. The key word is eventually, because initially you'll shed pounds and inches. At this point you're tangled in the web of the trap.

Your future is dismal. Your heritage is the reason.

A great many of us are descendants of famine survivors. Our bodies excel at constructing an energy reservoir by storing fat. When the body senses an energy reduction (through caloric deprivation) it protects us by slowing metabolism so that fat stores are maintained.

Metabolism is a very sensitive mechanism. Drastic reductions in caloric intake prompt your body to activate its starvation mode. The goal should be to make your body an efficient fat burner. You do this by increasing muscle mass to raise your basal metabolic rate (energy requirement at rest) and by decreasing your dietary calories sensibly.

Many women on my diet and exercise program find that they lose fat more efficiently on 1400 calories per day than they do on 1200 calories. The additional 200 calories per day assures that their bodies do not switch over to the starvation mode of preserving fat.

Each pound of muscle requires 75 calories per day for sustenance. That's why gaining muscle helps to supply a net calorie intake, and thus burns fat. Conversely, shrinking muscle lowers metabolic rate by approximately 75 calories per pound.

When your body begins cannibalizing muscle because it's starved for food calories, you're in a downward spiral. Fat delivers a metabolic load also. But it's only two calories per pound. You can rid yourself of 37.5 pounds of fat and not lower your metabolic rate any more than losing just one pound of muscle would cause.

Another web of the liquid-diet trap is the feeling that you can shift into a sensible approach once you've quickly dropped an initial amount of weight. Rarely does this work. Two factors stand in the way.

First, your drastic diet has enabled you to shed pounds without forming new habits that can be sustained long term. Forming sustainable new habits is very difficult. You wasted your prime motivation period on a liquid-diet trap that is very low in calories. Second, your metabolism is out of whack. If your body is used to 1500 calories per day, giving it 500 means it will be storing a pound of fat per week for some time. You'll quickly get discouraged with your sensible approach.

If you're now tangled in this drastic low-calorie trap, you should indeed switch to a sound approach. You will, however, have to weather a fat-storing storm until your metabolic rate adjusts itself. How long that takes depends on the degree of damage.

5

Solid Eating Habits Are Better Than Liquid Diets

Nothing hampers a fun occasion more insidiously than calorie worry. That ugly conflict between your fat-loss goals and your thirst for well-deserved enjoyment is the frustration of adult living in modern America.

Whether it's a picnic, a luncheon, restaurant dining or a family get-together, concern over calorie intake is aggravation you don't think you need.

We are constant decision makers: the beneficiaries of good ones, and the victims of poor ones.

Is fruit salad, a grilled skinless chicken breast, corn on the cob, and water really going to ruin your picnic? Or is fried chicken or a couple of hot dogs with baked beans and potato chips and lots of beer or wine coolers worth the extra pounds, inches and possible health deterioration?

This is the crux of our dilemma—the constant choices of how to nourish our bodies as measured against taste bud enjoyment and the psychological bond with eating.

Take heart. This problem can be solved.

Our daily eating habits need more attention, more preparation and more planning. They do not need low-calorie mixes to be used as meal replacements for sporadic weight loss followed by a joyous return to the same old over-indulgent eating patterns.

Review this checklist:

♦ Have you trimmed the fat from your favorite family recipes? This can usually be accomplished without sacrificing taste.

♦ Do you know the best choices at your favorite dining establishment? When selecting a restaurant, it helps to think in terms of what you want to eat instead of where you want to go.

♦ Do you know the calories in alcoholic beverages, including the mixers, and the impaired judgment that results from its consumption, along with any munchies you're tempted to include in the experience? Lost of fun calories here that you'll pay for later.

♦ Do you know the importance of eating less more often—several small eating episodes per day instead of one mammoth meal? Large meals increase fat storage.

♦ Is your water intake at least sixteen 8-ounce glasses per day, and maybe as many as 26? Don't let the simplicity of this strategy fool you—water is a fat-loss phenomenon.

♦ Are you stocked up on low-calorie alternatives to your favorite high-calorie snacks? Remember, saving just 100 calories per day means 10 pounds per year.

♦ Do you plan social activities that involve physical exertion instead of those featuring sitting and snacking? An evening of push-ups might not be appealing, but a volleyball game, bike ride, set of tennis or walk can be enjoyable.

Create a renewed, vitality-filled you.

Calorie worry does not have to spoil your fun. You must, however, prepare yourself. Small fundamental changes add up to a big difference over time.

6

Riding the Waves of The Urge to Eat

There's a new sport you ought to try: urge surfing. There's no wet suit required, no surf board needed, and you don't even have to fight the crowd at the beach.

To be an urge surfer requires only a desire to control your calorie intake, to shed fat, reduce cholesterol, or cut sodium intake. The waves you'll be riding are the emotions that trigger excessive eating. An urge is like a wave. It formulates slowly, picks up momentum, comes to a crest, breaks, and subsides gently on the shore.

You might think urges come on like monsters that can be satisfied only by giving in, by submission, by eating. Caving in to an urge results in more urges, more often, with more inertia behind them. But if you ride the wave, if you let it crest and pass, it will weaken and splash onto shore. You'll become a good urge surfer, and the next one will be easier to ride.

The image of the urge surfer is the work of Dr. G. Alan Marlett and Dr. Judith Gordon, psychologists at the University of Washington, authors of *Relapse Prevention* (Guilford Press, 1985), who studied the factors associated with relapse in not only dieters but also in alcoholics, smokers, drug addicts and compulsive gamblers.

There will always be urges, especially with your eating habits—the urge for a second helping, a salty snack. The waves roll in most furiously during "high tide," meaning your high-risk situations.

Being a good surfer means that you can detect the oncoming wave in time to prepare for it. You then have to be able to ride it out. Both of these—seeing it coming and knowing how to get on top—make you a good urge surfer. One without the other results in a lot of wipe-outs.

Figure out your high-tide times by making a list of your high-risk situations. These will be readily apparent if you keep a food diary for several days. The patterns will clearly emerge.

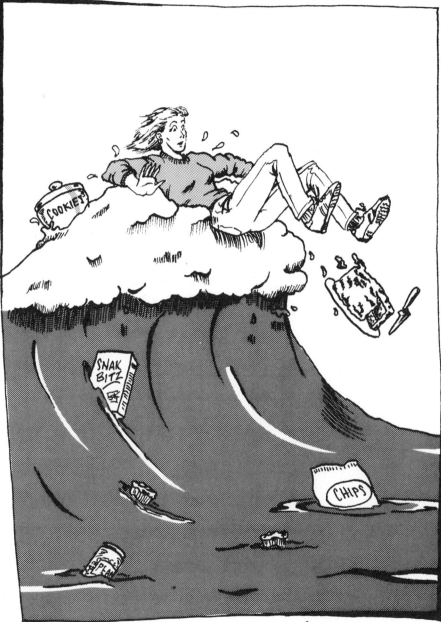

Learn to urge surf to control your appetite.

Are you at high risk when in the house alone, maybe just before the kids come home from school? Or, is it at night in front of the TV, subjected to a billion-dollar advertising industry unsurpassed at urging you to consume food? Are you a stress eater, using calories to douse the flames of frustration? Do you cope with boredom by pampering yourself with food you really don't need?

Ride the wave of urges by having a list of alternative activities to eating. This list might include such things as taking a walk, shopping, exercising, doing your fingernails, brushing your teeth, reading a fitness publication, taking a bath, taking a drive, refinishing furniture, working in the garden, painting, or imagining being in great shape. Refer to it often.

7

Getting to the Root of A Sweet Tooth

After a hearty meal, do you still need the taste of something sweet? Even when there is no possible way that your body could require nourishment, does a hefty slice of layer cake with two scoops of ice cream seem irresistible?

At the shopping mall, do you fall victim to the aromas of baking cookies or cinnamon pastries?

Does chocolate taste good any time?

If these descriptions fit, you probably think you're under the relentless control of a sweet tooth.

If a barrel of sweets is your idea of ecstasy, try drinking distilled water with loads of sugar poured in. If you find the sugar water to be the next best thing to seeing Saddam Hussein drown in the oil slick that he polluted the Persian Gulf with, then you've got a legitimate 100-percent sweet tooth.

But research shows that not many women craving sweets rush to the sugar bowl and empty it into a glass of water. Pies, cookies, candy bars and cakes are devoured in a feeding frenzy, however. And when you look closely at such foods, you realize that most of the calories in them come from fat—from shortening, oil, cream—not from sugar.

Sugar, which has never been proven to cause any harm other than tooth decay, delivers only four calories per gram. Fat is more than twice as potent.

So, do you have a sweet tooth, or a fat tooth?

Researchers at the University of Michigan several years ago decided to offer obese women plain fat, to which their reaction was even more negative than it was to sugar water.

The researchers, therefore, started combining sugar and fat to see how both obese women and women of normal weight reacted. They both took plain skim milk (no fat) and heavy cream (lots of fat) and started adding sugar to them.

"If you start adding sugar to skim milk, normal-weight women will like it better and better until you hit 5 to 10 percent sugar—after that it's too sweet. Fat women, on the other hand, will start calling it too sweet at only 4 percent sugar," reported Adam Drewnowski, Ph.D., one of the researchers.

"If you start adding sugar to heavy cream," continued Drewnowski, "normal-weight women will like the mixture up to 9 percent sugar. But fat women will like the same amount of sweetness even more. If you make it fattier, they'll love it."

So, fat women like plain sweetness less than normal-weight women, but they like sweetened fats a lot more.

Women who used to be fat but have lost weight are in double jeopardy—they like both. This may be one reason why the vast majority regain their lost body fat.

Our sweet tooth takes in a lot of dietary fat. This perhaps explains why sugar substitutes, which have been in our food supply for years, have not trimmed our waistlines.

Having made this distinction, how can you put it to use?

♦ Try Entenmann's fat-free baked goods (yellow banner on the box).

♦ Switch from ice cream to ice milk, frozen yogurt, or Toffuti.

♦ Give products made with fake fat—such as Simple Pleasures—a try.

The cravings we've traditionally identified as the existence of a sweet tooth are doomed to continue. Fortunately, food makers are wringing saturated fat out of many foods, even french fries and hamburgers.

Besides Simple Pleasures, more foods will be coming out that are made with low-calorie fat substitutes, which have been undergoing research for years.

We need more products in restaurants and on grocery shelves that offer a creamy, textured taste with a zing of sweetness but not the calorie load of dietary fat.

Our sweet-fat tooth needs some low-calorie satisfaction.

8

Seven Ways to Avoid Sweets

From rum cake to truffles to chocolate chip cookies, 'tis the season to be baking. Sweets, which are usually a combination of simple sugar and dietary fat, are everywhere.

We're indulging, aren't we?

During the season to be jolly, we're operating under the nutritional equivalent of "But now, no payments until January." Dietary discipline is fully suspended, as readily as financial concerns are jettisoned along the MasterCard/Visa fast track. The credit-card mentality affects our waistlines as much as our pocketbooks.

If your sweet tooth is a cavern about the size of the Grand Canyon, here are a few things you can do to keep from running excessive calorie charges.

♦ **Use opaque containers.**
Clear wrap is deadly. The more often you have to go eyeball-to-triglyceride with your favorite sweet, the more it ends up in your mouth. Opaque containers in inconvenient storage places reduce impulsive binges.

♦ **Don't miss a square meal.**
Skipping a meal so you can indulge in a 1000-calorie baked good is kind of like your kid dropping out of college to buy a Jaguar. It's a brief thrill with severe consequences down the road.

It's especially important to integrate firm meals with shopping-mall excursions.

♦ **Carry an insulated water bottle.**
Drown your sweet cravings. Water is a terrific appetite regulator. Carry a 32-ounce insulated water bottle—you know, the kind with the screw-on lid and straw—wherever you go. Sip on water continually throughout the day.

♦ **At the office, try to avoid the "sweets buffet."**
Quarantine the room that houses the dazzling display of home-baked

goodies. If the room is essential to your employment, try to have the sweets moved, or organize your workload to minimize trips into the room. If it's right next to the coffee—and you've got to have coffee—pack your own thermos until the calorie assault ceases.

♦ **Remember to urge-surf.**
Think of a craving as a wave building in the ocean. Try to see it coming as much in advance as possible. You've got to know how to get over it instead of letting it crash over you. You'll wipe out a few times, but you'll get better with practice.

♦ **Refine your grocery list.**
Make up for the fact that you'll be nipping at the specialties of the season by leaving behind the cookies, chips, and crackers that normally find their way into your grocery cart. Make whatever you "must have for the kids" something that is not your overwhelming temptation.

♦ **Watch only essential television programs.**
TV exposes us to a billion-dollar advertising that knows how to prompt us to eat. It has its fingers on all our impulse buttons. Research shows time and again that fatter people spend more time in front of the tube. Limit your exposure by selecting TV viewing that is essential.

We've pampered ourselves with excessive holiday sweets a long time. It's an American tradition, one that contributes to bulging waistlines, declining health, accelerated aging, and fitness frustration.

Isn't it about time you took control of your sweet tooth?

These seven changes can help keep your eyes, and your appetite, headed in the right direction.

9

Try These Calorie Busters to Stay Slim

Do you want a simple concept to combat calorie exposure?
Keep these four words in mind: *Cereal, salad, soup,* and *fruit.*

These are your allies. Used correctly, they'll guide you through the holiday fat-gaining season and deliver you into your future years in slimness.

Here's how it works.

Cereal signifies a breakfast of one to two ounces of any of the several nutritious cold cereals currently available. Fiber One, Cheerios, Shredded Wheat, Frosted Mini Wheats, and Heartwise are among the dozen or so that deliver approximately 110 calories per ounce, with a fair shake of vitamins and fiber. Douse in skim milk, preferably.

If your taste buds aren't ready for fatless milk, descend the fat-content ladder one step at a time: from whole milk to 2 percent to 1 percent to skim.

In place of a cold cereal, you could eat ¾ cup of cooked oatmeal, spiced with cinnamon, nutmeg, and maybe even a banana.

Don't let the simplicity of the cereal suggestion cause you to overlook it.

If you're going to maintain slimness and good health, you must start your day with a wholesome breakfast. Too many of us mistakenly skip this important meal, believing we're saving calories. We'll only overeat later. Research studies clearly show the advantages of spreading calories throughout the day, as opposed to saving up for one big food fest.

Putting cereal into your belly each morning will enable you to bypass the offerings of sweets around the coffee table at the office.

Make salad and/or soup the main courses of every lunch and dinner over which you have control. This especially includes shopping mall junkets. You can find salad almost everywhere.

Watch out for so-called salad bars that are really mega-calorie mine fields. An effective guideline is to restrict yourself to using the tongs—no ladle. If you have to scoop something, you can bet it's loaded with a high-calorie oil or mayonnaise. Anything that drips—even marinated vegetables—should be avoided or used sparingly.

You can find plenty of dressings that offer no more than eight calories per tablespoon. Buy a Weight Watchers' dressing to keep in your purse or pocket in case the restaurant can't accommodate you.

Always order salad dressing on the side. Instead of drowning your salad in it, dip the tines of your fork into the dressing before you spear your salad. In this way you'll use just enough to deliver the taste.

Remember salad when you're at the shopping mall being overwhelmed by the aromas of cinnamon and chocolate chips. A salad will give you more sustainable energy for your shopping excursion and less body fat to deal with later.

Soup is the salad alternative. Find a good, low-calorie, low-sodium soup recipe. Take a couple of hours some Sunday afternoon to make a gigantic potful of this hearty soup. Dispense it into freezer bags to use for several weeks.

Sodium is the culprit in most soups. Be careful of what you order in a restaurant. You want a blend of spices and not salt.

An arsenal of fruit should stand ready to satisfy snack impulses. Make a vow to abandon high-calorie goodies. Our body's cells deal more efficiently with fruit than with cookies, cakes, and candies.

Don't let yourself get hungry—grab an apple, orange or banana.

Remember: *cereal, salad, soup,* and *fruit.*

There'll be plenty of social occasions where you overdose on hors d'oeuvres, prime rib, and pecan pie. To counteract these suspensions in dietary discipline, make a vow to yourself.

Cereal, salad, soup, and *fruit.*

10

Break Your String of Yo-Yo Dieting

Sometime between every Thanksgiving and Christmas, do you tell yourself that right after the first of the year you're going to get into shape? Then you decide to wait until after the Super Bowl, because everyone overeats during this final football weekend.

Before you know it, it's almost the end of February and you still haven't taken the next step. Or maybe you start a program and then become complacent.

It's estimated that 65 million Americans have weight reduction at the top of their list of New Year's resolutions. It's unclear, however, as to how many abandon the idea.

Yo-yo dieting is very common. If you overeat compulsively, you'll probably also diet compulsively. You merely move from one cycle to the other. To achieve long-term success, you must determine if you are suppressing food at the moment or learning to control it.

Suppressing food is like painting over rust. It might look good for a while, but soon the rust will bleed through while continuing to spread. "Diet" usually means suppressing food. For a while, you can deny yourself. But it won't take long for the novelty to wear off.

Controlling food means giving it a well-defined role in your life—nourishment. It's not amusement, a companion, nor a stress-relief valve. You eat when you're hungry, and you stop eating when you're no longer hungry.

In *Diets Don't Work,* Bob Schwartz claims that fat people eat until they are full or until the food on the plate is all gone. Naturally thin people, he says, eat until they are no longer hungry.

Have you ever been seated at the dinner table about halfway through a meal and been interrupted by a phone call or a visitor? Several minutes later you return to the table, and looking down at the food you had planned to eat you realize you're no longer hungry.

If not for the interruption you would have eaten several hundred more calories, taking your appetite meter past "not hungry" and all the way to "full."

Schwartz also wants us to play with our food. Playing with it reduces the reverence we extend to food and the power we give it over ourselves. Eating is the pre-eminent pastime in the American culture. That's why we're always battling the bulges.

The other part of the slimness equation is exercise. Effective exercise is an arduous task, but the feeling you get from doing it becomes an addiction. I call it the adrenaline fix. I have to have a fix every forty-eight to seventy-two hours.

If you don't know what I mean by adrenaline fix, you're probably only exerting, not really exercising. Exercise is a strategy to bring about physiological improvement. Too many people think of any motion, or inducement of perspiration or soreness as exercise. And others do such easy workouts that they're merely amusing themselves.

Control your calorie intake and push past the threshold point of exercise and you can make this year the year you master a fitness lifestyle.

11

Water Aids in Weight Loss

Studies have shown a relationship between water intake and fat deposits: the more water the less fat, and the less water the more fat.

The reason? The kidneys are unable to function without adequate water. When they do not work to capacity some of their load is dumped onto

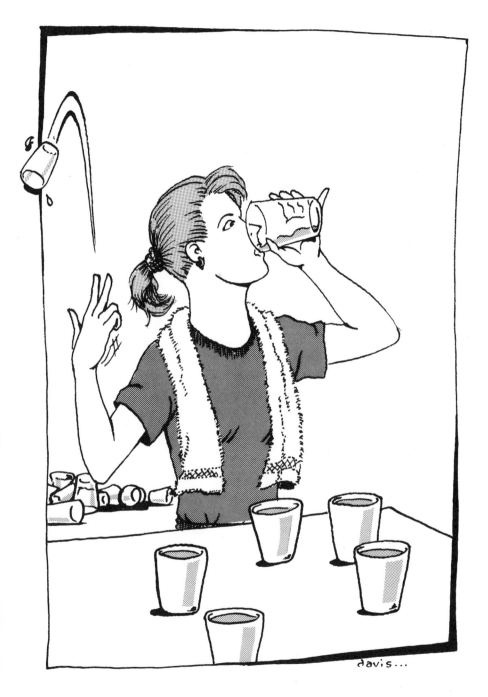

". . . 11 glasses down and only 5 to go!"

the liver. This diverts the liver from its primary function, which is to metabolize stored fat into usable energy. Because it's performing the chores of the water-depleted kidneys, the liver metabolizes less fat.

Overeating can also be averted through water intake, as water can keep the stomach feeling full and satisfied between meals, thus preventing it from signaling the brain that it is hungry. When water is consumed in conjunction with foods high in fiber, this satiated feeling increases because the fiber in these foods actually absorbs the water and swells in size.

The standard recommendation is a minimum of eight glasses per day, a total of sixty-four ounces. It's also advisable to include one glass just before each meal, and one during each meal. But new research shows that it's beneficial to drink even more water.

Most of the dieters in my Nautilus Diet programs consume sixteen glasses of water a day. Some even work up to thirty-two glasses, or two gallons a day!

The participants who drink the most water tend to lose the most fat.

If you are serious about losing fat, I recommend that you purchase a plastic water bottle, the kind with a built-in straw, readily available in supermarkets, service stations, and convenience stores. With such a bottle you can carry water with you throughout the day for continuous drinking.

For best results the water should be ice cold. A gallon of cold water (40 degrees Fahrenheit) requires 226 calories of heat energy to warm it to core body temperature (98.6 degrees Fahrenheit).

Furthermore, water is very important to an exercise program; it gives muscles their natural ability to contract and prevent dehydration as well. Water also helps to prevent sagging skin that usually follows significant fat loss.

Drink even if you're not thirsty. Responding to thirst will prevent only severe dehydration. It will not prompt you to drink the water you need to function at your peak.

Other than herbal tea, liquids containing water are not adequate substitutes for it. Coffee, soft drinks, iced tea, and even so-called sports drinks or energy drinks contain other chemicals that negate or offset the benefits of pure water. However, a sprig of mint or slice of lemon is okay for flavoring.

Inadequate water causes the body to perceive a threat to survival, and thus it begins to hold on to every drop. Water is then stored outside the cells, showing up as swollen feet, legs, or hands, in what we commonly refer to as water retention.

The best way to overcome water retention is to give your body the water it needs. Only then will stored water be released.

Restricting your water intake makes you constipated. When deprived of water your system pulls it from your lower intestines and bowel, thus creating hard dry stools. Water helps rid the body of waste, which is more critical during periods of fat reduction since metabolized fat must be shed.

Begin your water-drinking program with eight 8-ounce glasses, or two quarts of ice cold water each day for the first week. Increase this by one glass per day until you get to sixteen 8-ounce glasses, or one gallon a day.

If possible, gradually work up to a daily consumption of twenty-four 8-ounce glasses of water. Your system will thank you for it, and you'll soon be rewarded with a leaner, stronger body.

12

Try Where/When/How Diet Plan

If your efforts to control what you eat are failing miserably, try instead restricting where, when and how you consume calories. Deny yourself nothing; just enjoy food only in the appropriate place, at the proper time, and in the correct way.

Make an effort to master the following three-point method. This might be only a snail's pace to slimness, but small change compounds its benefit over the long haul.

♦ **Where? In only one place**.
Do you eat in front of the television? Do you munch a snack in the bedroom, or on the porch? Do you enjoy lunch at your desk in the office?

What you eat and how much you eat are affected by the manner in which you eat.

There should be one place in the home where you consume food, and it should be the only place you do so. Likewise at work—eat in just one place. Furthermore, you should do nothing else in this place. If it's a kitchen table, for instance, do not sit at it to read the newspaper, play cards, or help the kids with homework.

The danger in eating anywhere and everywhere in the house or office is that you will then tend to feel hungry while in those places. It isn't really hunger, however, it's probably just appetite. It can even be a nervous habit.

♦ **When? On a planned schedule.**

Impulsive binges can be disastrous. Winging it with regard to your daily food intake is like spending money without first budgeting it.

You should have a plan, a schedule. It should contain as much detail as possible—time, place, and what you are to eat.

A schedule does not necessarily mean three meals a day at conventional times. You should develop a schedule that's convenient for you, one that you can follow.

Following a schedule will help you eat less and think more. It will help you conquer urges by waiting them out, waiting until your next scheduled meal or snack.

♦ **How? Do nothing else while you eat.**

Combining eating with watching TV, talking on the phone, reading a magazine, or any other activity poses two distinct disadvantages.

The first is that it pairs eating with another activity. Just out of habit the event can stimulate appetite. You'll be more apt to feel hungry during these other activities that you associate with eating.

The second disadvantage is that you won't be entirely conscious of your food consumption. Calories should be tasted.

If implementing this three-point plan seems awkward and difficult, that's a sure sign you need it. My bet is that, overall, you'll eat fewer calories if you use the proper eating procedures.

13

The Drastically Low Calorie Trap

In 1990, when Oprah Winfrey fasted her way to slimness, I predicted that she'd gain back all she'd lost. The "Drastically Low Calorie Trap," I called it.

Oprah's joy ride with slimness was soon over. On her show in November of the same year, she vowed to "never diet again," and later added, "I'll certainly never fast again."

Ultimately, OptiFast failed Oprah. She termed her show's topic, "The Pain of the Regain."

After the holidays, your clothes seem to mysteriously shrink, you become disgusted with yourself, and the holiday party is over. In this desperate state, you're ripe for an Oprahlike diet disaster.

Reports have it that Slim Fast advertising will total roughly $100 million this year, and it should continue to dominate the billion-dollar meal-replacement market.

Seizing upon your desperation—your willingness to believe there's a quick and easy solution—many diet methods will compete for your attention.

So, what are you mixing in your blender that you're calling a meal?

As boring as this may sound, look for something sensible. There are no great breakthroughs that have any validity. Two pounds per week is the maximum fat-loss that will last. Increase your energy expenditure through exercise and set up a balanced eating plan that provides at least 1000 calories per day.

The average-size man can probably lose weight on 2000 calories per day, and the average-size woman about 1400. Distribute the calories: 60 percent carbohydrate, 20 percent fat and 20 percent protein.

Saturated fat should be restricted to 10 percent of your total calories. Up to another 10 percent should be composed of unsaturated fats.

Saturated fats are contained in animal products—red meat, lard, butter, poultry with skin, and whole milk dairy products. Two vegetable oils, palm and coconut, are also highly saturated.

Unsaturated fats are found primarily in vegetable oils. They are foods that are liquid at room temperature.

If you need to know this distinction in more detail, there are plenty of books at the library and in bookstores that will assist you.

Saturated fat and a sedentary lifestyle are severe health hazards. Stanford and Southern California medical researchers say this combination accounts for as much as 60 percent of the colon/rectal cancer rates in men and 40 percent of the cancer rates in women.

Your eating and exercising habits are important enough to merit time and effort.

The International Journal of Obesity reported recently that yo-yo dieting changes the fat distribution in women and increases health risks. Yale researchers found that yo-yo dieters showed greater amounts of adipose (fat) tissue above the waist than below the waist, when compared to women who've never dieted. Fat from above the waist is either a cause or an indication of increased risk of heart disease or cancer.

Traditionally, January is diet month because it follows the holiday season. Ninety-five percent of those who diet to lose weight gain it back, simply because their methods were austere and impractical for the long term.

If you want results that last, think not in terms of diet but of a sensible eating plan and regular exercise.

Oprah wishes she had.

14

Listing Goals Is Write Way to Lose Weight

Maybe you've recently arrived at the point of being fed up and disgusted with your physical contour and physical condition. Thus, you passionately resolve: shape up or die!

Food becomes your enemy, sweat your savior. You'll get thin quickly and never be fat again!

If this describes you, turn off your Jane Fonda tape and try to let reason infiltrate the mayhem of your mind.

Millions of frustrated dieters go up and down, pursuing an elusive ideal. Within a year 95 percent regain all they've lost.

Desperation doesn't work.

But goals do. A written, specific, step-by-step, detailed, thoughtful plan can remedy the aggravation that overwhelms you.

Here is what you do.

♦ Describe—in writing—the way you want to be in six months, one year, and five years. This statement should include such things as the size and style of clothing you will wear; things you'll do that maybe you're avoiding now; and the confidence you'll feel and exhibit, and what that will add to your life.

Knowing your outcome is the first key to reaching it. The more detail, the better. Be sure to use at least three points in the future.

♦ Write down your reasons for your goals. Maybe you want to look better, feel great, have more energy, or excel at a sport.

Why is your goal important, where does it rank, and how does it fit in with other goals?

If you have enough reasons you can do anything. Reasons are the difference between merely being interested and being totally committed to an objective.

♦ List at least seven resources that will help you attain all three tiers of your goal. This may include your personal character traits, spouse support, a book or motivational material, professional counseling or guidance.

♦ Ask yourself "What prevents me from already having what I desire?" Search your soul for reasons and write them down. If you think you can't achieve your goals, ask yourself, "But what would happen if I could?" Search out a detailed answer to each question.

♦ Have the flexibility to keep at it until it happens. Adjustments are going to be necessary. When the mind has a defined target, it can focus and direct and refocus and redirect until it reaches the intended goal.

Start writing things down—now. A study of 1953 Yale graduates showed twenty years later that the 3 percent with written goals had a combined net worth that exceeded the 97 percent who did not commit their goals to writing upon graduation.

This is not an automatic process, but it is a very successful one.

15

Dieting Takes More Than Just Counting Fat

Perhaps you're like the woman who chooses the food she eats based on only one criterion—total grams of fat. There are cookies, cakes, and frozen desserts that are very much like ice cream that have significantly reduced or eliminated fat, thanks to some innovative substitutes.

It is becoming vogue, this idea of monitoring dietary fat and running wild with carbohydrates and proteins. Sweet lovers, rejoice! Into every celebration, however, there seems to be a guy who sneezes on the fat-free pastries. While limiting fat intake is a forceful step in the right direction, there is grave danger of it backfiring.

Calories still count. Before the dawning of fat substitutes, limiting fat could be counted on to bring about a corresponding reduction in calories.

Studies do indeed show that dietary fat sticks to the ribs of obese people disproportionately when compared with the same number of calories from protein and carbohydrate. But don't think you can eat all the bananas you want, and for sure don't go wild with fake-fat baked goods. Your total calories could climb astronomically.

If you're eating a low-fat, high-calorie diet, you're in uncharted waters. Until and unless clinical research supports the notion that carbohydrate and protein don't find their way into fat cells, you'd be wise to hold calories in check.

A calorie is a unit of energy, and what our bodies don't immediately need they store. Fat is simply a great-tasting concentrated package of calories.

"Preferences for high-fat foods may involve both body and mind as well as cultural factors. There is evidence that some of our food preferences are under metabolic as well as psychological control. Cultural factors also play a major role. Some food habits are acquired in early childhood and others are dictated by social norms.

"Recent societal changes, including an increased pace of life, have made high-fat foods a staple of the American diet. The net result is that the combination of fat tooth preferences and a fat-rich environment has produced deeply rooted eating habits that are remarkably resistant to change."

That statement was made by Adam Drewnowski, director of the Program in Human Nutrition at the University of Michigan. It was published in the foreword of *Controlling Your Fat Tooth* by Joseph C. Piscatella (Workman Publishing, 1991).

Brain chemistry can dictate a strong craving for fatty foods. With all of our awareness of the dangers of high-fat diets, our overall reduction is slight, says Piscatella.

His book states:

◆ Since 1980, we've cut down on red meat, whole milk, and butter. But we're now eating more saturated fat.

◆ We eat 33 billion hamburgers a year, about three per week for every person in the country.

◆ Women have cut down on red meat, but consumption among males has remained steady.

◆ Females get their fat from margarine, dairy foods, mayonnaise, and salad dressings.

◆ We're eating the same amount of ice cream as in 1980, but the fat content has soared because of the popularity of brands like Haagen-Dazs, Ben & Jerry's, and Frusen Gladje.

◆ Hard cheese consumption has doubled since 1968. We're eating it most in cheeseburgers and pizzas.

- We're eating more fats and oils, commercially baked goods and snack foods. Croissants, a particularly fatty bakery item, has become a super-market staple.

- Sales of commercial cheesecakes are at record levels.

- Candy consumption has risen.

Eating too much dietary fat is the most significant reason for the dra-matic increase in diet-induced diseases in North America, particularly heart disease, cancer, and obesity.

Piscatella's book can help you set up a fat-budgeting system for select-ing food at home, in a supermarket, or at a restaurant. Following such ad-vice is a better strategy than counting grams of fat and ignoring calories.

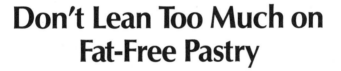

Don't Lean Too Much on Fat-Free Pastry

Fat-free pastries are a wonderful invention of the final decade of the twentieth century—maybe. History will record it so, only if we do not abuse the opportunity for overall higher-quality eating habits.

We stand the chance to keep the fat off our bodies with less resentment from our taste buds. But don't think that adipose tissue will become a thing of the past without any effort on our part.

Here's what is happening.

Fat-free pastries are found in the Entenmann's boxes with the yellow banners. Bunge Foods also supplies fat-free mixes for food companies and local bakeries, so that we can have our cake and remain fatless, too.

A host of other fat-free baked goods are soon to be available, ready to take the guilt out of our indulgence.

Eliminating the fat hasn't sacrificed any taste in most of these products. They also do not rely on fat substitutes or any other unusual ingredients.

The first fat-reducing step was to replace whole eggs with egg whites and whole milk with skim. Then these bakers changed the proportions and combinations of starches, gums, and emulsifiers, making it possible to eliminate shortening and oils.

To compensate for the loss of the fat flavor, however, more sugar is added.

The labels on these products list such things as:

♦ Emulsifiers such as lecithin and mono- and diglycerides for softness and uniform texture;

♦ Starches and gums (gums are actually a type of dietary fiber) for thickness;

♦ Humectants such as propylene and glycol for moistness.

With so much to cheer about, what's keeping us from starting the parade?

First, you've got to remember total calories. Fat-free provides leeway for a greater daily calorie total, perhaps, but don't stop counting.

Second, most of us need to upgrade our daily nutritional intake in ways other than simply reducing dietary fat. We also need more fruits, whole grains, and vegetables. A fat-free Danish is no substitute for whole-grain cereal.

Third, these fat-free products carry higher price tags. The health improvement, however, is worth not being cheap.

Fat-free products pose a tasty option. Just don't be thinking that the only dietary guideline that matters is to select the boxes with the yellow banners. If you crowd out the fruits, vegetables, and whole grains, dietary fat reduction will prove counter-productive.

17

Bread-and-Butter Facts About Fat

There is much we can learn from the recent death of football player Lyle Alzado, but it isn't about the hazards of muscle-building chemicals. While those are prevalent in locker rooms, most of us are not tempted to boost our testosterone level. If ever we were, the brain cancer that afflicted Alzado should scare us straight.

For those who fail to commit Sunday afternoons to football fanaticism, Alzado was once a prominent gridiron warrior who attempted a post-retirement comeback in 1990. He relied on steroids his entire career and

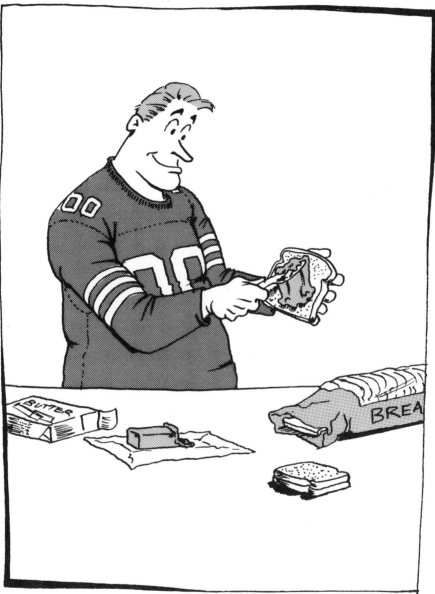

Keep your butter intake to a minimum.

then added human growth hormone injections in preparation for his failed comeback attempt.

The man fights for his life and loses, and if we use Alzado's tragedy only to disdain artificial muscle fertilizer, we've missed something far more applicable.

We're ingesting chemicals that are surely killing us, too, though the process may be more insidious. We've deflected the warnings about as often as Alzado ignored tales of shriveled testicles and racing heart-beats.

Too much saturated dietary fat makes life's journey short and bumpy. If a sedentary lifestyle is also involved, then it's even shorter and bumpier.

Even though it seems our sanity is at stake in keeping track of all the conflicting messages, the best evidence demands that no more than 10 percent of our daily calories should be supplied by the likes of beef, butter, poultry, and three vegetable oils that reside in many processed snack foods: palm, palm kernel, and coconut.

Saturated fat produces cholesterol in our coronary arteries, restricting oxygen flow to the heart. Actual cholesterol intake from food (animal's liver) also mucks up the pipeline.

One out of five males in this country suffers a heart attack by age sixty. Cheeseburgers, milkshakes, and doughnuts are helping half of us die from blood vessel disease. Twice as many women die from cardiovascular disease than from all other types of cancer. The daily death toll is 2000 Americans. Countries without such an addiction to saturated fat have considerably lower rates of heart failure.

If Lyle Alzado was ill-advised to bulk up through chemical aids, aren't we equally ill-advised to eat foods that slowly suffocate our hearts? Besides, we gain no fame or fortune from our daily fat intake.

Two other forms of dietary fat—polyunsaturated and monoun-saturated—may actually reduce cholesterol. It would be dangerous, how-ever, to consider them antidotes to saturated fat overload. The reason for this is both the danger of obesity and that other great killer—cancer.

Thirty-five types of cancer, including breast, colon, and prostate, do not differentiate types of fat; they simply feed on all three.

Polyunsaturated fats include safflower, soybean, sunflower, corn, cottonseed, and sesame oils. Monounsaturated oils include olive, canola, peanut, avocado, and nut. You'll have to read the food labels to detect these ingredients.

The more liquid a fat becomes at room temperature, the less saturated it is. That's why margarine is less damaging than butter. Consumption of polyunsaturated fat and monounsaturated fat should each be restricted to

10 percent of daily calorie total, too, just like saturated fat. Added together, this would make a diet that is no more than 30 percent fat.

It's estimated that the typical American registers 37 percent of his or her calories per day from fat. Reducing total dietary fat intake reduces cancer risk—it's that simple.

Greater detail on fat and its hiding places in so many of the foods we love is provided in many books. One that gives a strong account of the situation along with 200 recipes for low-fat eating is *Controlling Your Fat Tooth,* by Joseph C. Piscatella.

In its proper dosage, dietary fat serves useful purposes in the body. For one thing, fat delivers vitamins A, D, E, and K into the cells. Fat is necessary. The goal is to control it not to eliminate it.

The problem is that we are in love with the taste of fat, especially if it is sweetened.

If we would control our daily calories, and allocate 10 percent to each of the fats, we'd live longer and healthier. Don't be so alarmed that you aren't sensible. Try to identify your daily fat consumption and whittle it down to 10 percent of total calories of each kind.

Think of this when Lyle Alzado's death tugs at your heart and confounds your mind.

18

We're Slow to Appreciate Fast Foods

Burgers, french fries, pizzas, potato chips, and shakes. These are foods Americans love to eat.

They're also foods that Americans feel guilty about—guilty because many consumer activists state that such foods have no redeeming nutritional qualities.

Television advertising always pictures fast foods in a fun-filled family atmosphere that makes them seem wholesome, nutritious and all-American. What's the fitness-minded individual to do? Can you eat fast foods without feeling guilty? Or should you avoid them altogether?

Judith Stern and R.V. Denenberg evaluated fast-food meals according to the U.S. Recommended Daily Allowances for vitamins and minerals. These three meals are representative:

♦ Fried chicken (three pieces), roll, coleslaw, potatoes.

♦ Half of a 10-inch pizza, iced tea with two spoons of sugar.

♦ Fried fish sandwich, regular order of fries, vanilla shake.

The three fast-food meals are a good source of vitamin B-1 (thiamine), B-2, and niacin. If fortified milk products are consumed, the meals would also be adequate for children's needs for vitamin D. The meals tend to be low in vitamin A, B-6, folacin, pantothenic acid, and C. But with appropriate food choices for the rest of the day, the proper levels can be reached. For example, you should consume green and yellow vegetables in your other meals.

Fast foods have ample supplies of calcium, phosphorus, sodium, iodine, and zinc. Pizza is especially high in calcium because of the cheese. Most fast foods, however, lack concentrations of the following minerals: copper, iron, magnesium, and manganese. To supply these missing nutrients, it would be wise to consume green leafy vegetables, fruits, nuts, and occasionally liver at other meals.

The average fast-food meal contains about 25 grams of protein. This amounts to 46 percent of a man's and 56 percent of a woman's daily needs.

Shakes and cola drinks contain an abundance of calories. Shakes that are made with skim milk, or an appreciable amount of fat-free milk solids, would add protein and calcium to the meal. The only nutrients in cola drinks are water and carbohydrates.

Scientific research shows that the American public has the safest, the most abundant, the most nutritious, and the most economical supply of food that any people have ever had. Yet, it is also the most misunderstood food supply of all time.

What the American people need is nutrition education. Nutrition education should be based on respect of all foods. Whether food is termed fast, traditional, or homemade, the same principles of balance and moderation apply.

19

How to Cut Fast-Food Calories

Fast food doesn't have to be the fast track to fatness. Mayonnaise lovers, however, are in for a struggle. The taste buds also have to spurn cheese specialty and full-strength salad dressings.

Not to be discarded, however, is the plain hamburger. It contains only about 300 calories. That includes lettuce, tomato, and bun. It's the extra meat and the juicy stuff that oozes out the sides of your mouth that escalates calories.

The mayo on a McDLT contains more calories (135) than a small order of french fries. Mayo contributes 150 calories to the Burger King Whopper and 200 to BK's Chicken Specialty.

The tartar sauce on a McDonald's Filet-o-Fish sandwich packs 16 grams of fat and 144 calories. The specialty sauce on the BK broiler has 90 calories.

Whether sliced onto a burger, cooked into a pizza, or melted onto a baked potato, most cheeses offer a high concentration of calories and saturated fat.

That means baked potatoes perhaps spiced with pepper or lemon but otherwise plain. Such a maneuver extricates 306 calories at Wendy's.

Order pizza with cheese on only half. You can accomplish this at Pizza Hut by requesting a hand-tossed pepperoni pizza without the pepperoni. Huh? It's automatically made with only half the cheese of a cheese pizza.

A lite vinaigrette or reduced-calorie Italian salad dressing may save you 100 calories per salad.

A sensible breakfast at McDonald's would mean an Apple Bran Muffin, English muffin, Cheerios, or Wheaties. If you want hot cakes, go easy on the syrup and butter, which contain one-third of the calories and two-thirds of the fat.

For a snack or dessert under the golden arches, restrict yourself to a frozen yogurt, orange sorbet, or a low-fat shake.

Burger King's Chicken Tenders should be dipped into barbecue, honey, or sweet and sour sauce instead of ranch or tartar.

At the Wendy's Super Bar, reach for the tortillas, beans, rice, and pasta rather than the tacos, meat, and garlic toast. Or, order a fish fillet or chili.

A well-balanced Arby's meal would consist of a French Dip Roast Beef Sandwich (one-third less fat than regular roast beef), plain baked potato and side salad with light Italian dressing.

Do Kentucky Fried Chicken right by enjoying two pieces of corn on the cob, and one piece of chicken—skinless. In fried chicken, you see, saturated fat is most skin deep. That's why extra crispy is 45 percent fattier than the Colonel's original recipe. And if you're tempted to order French fries, mashed potatoes with gravy are less than half the calories.

Most franchise operations will provide nutritional information on request, even if that means writing to the home office. Another pointer for enacting these suggestions is to use the drive-through window so you won't be tempted by the aromas of fattier foods.

Space does not permit me to specify selections at some other popular chains. You should be able to extrapolate from this sampling.

Before long your taste buds won't even like mayonnaise.

20

What's Good About Fast Foods

Several years ago I sent my updated nutrition book to Howard Appledorf, a food science professor at the University of Florida. In Chapter one, I discussed the optimum diet for health and fitness: 59 percent carbohydrates, 28 percent fats, and 13 percent proteins.

While reviewing my book, Appledorf made an unexpected comparison.

He had just finished extensive nutrient analyses of fast foods. One of the most popular fast-food meals (a hamburger, french fries, and a shake) was evaluated at 59 percent carbohydrates, 28 percent fats, and 13 percent proteins—identical to the optimum diet for health and fitness.

"No one who has a basic knowledge of nutrition should really be surprised at that," the professor insisted to me. "A hamburger dinner is loaded with carbohydrates from bread, potatoes, milk, and sugar.

"And there's at least one serving from each of the Basic Four food groups, so it is well-balanced nutritionally. Hamburgers, french fries, and shakes make a valuable contribution to a person's nutritional status." (It should be noted that Appledorf was referring to a regular, small-size McDonald's hamburger, the 70-cent variety, not the Big Mac or Quarter Pounder.)

A hamburger meal couldn't be that nutritious, I thought to myself as I pored over the data. I found what I considered to be an important deficiency. "Your nutrient analyses," I said, "reveal that a hamburger dinner is low in vitamin A, and that's not good."

"But," Appledorf smiled, "if a consumer uses ketchup on his french fries, he has sufficient vitamin A."

He handed me additional data, which included ketchup on the french fries, to prove his point.

I learned something about fast foods that day, and I gained a special

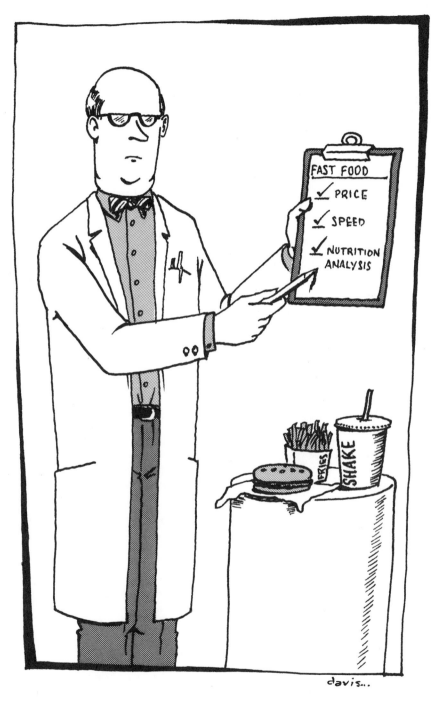

Analyses show that many fast foods are surprisingly nutritious.

appreciation for fast-food hamburgers. Since then I've been involved in much fast-food research on my own, and I'd like to share some of the facts with you.

How popular are fast foods?

Of the 50 million Americans who eat out daily, more than a quarter choose fast food. Statistics show the average adult eats in a fast-food restaurant nine times a month.

Although the popularity of fast foods is increasing, so is criticism. Critics say that fast food is notoriously high in sugar, fat, calories, and salt, while low in fiber.

What the critics do not point out is that fast food refers to a generic category of food prepared and served in rapid order. Fast refers to service rather than food.

The ultimate fast food is human milk. When an infant cries, the mother will nurse. Human milk is high in calories, fat, and sugar, and low in fiber. But no one criticizes it as being hazardous to the infant's health.

Why do Americans like fast food?

The popularity of fast-food restaurants seems to be tied to society's preoccupation with speed and security.

The speed at which food is selected and served has become important to the worker. At noon, workers from a factory or office begin an efficient trek to the burger shop. The ordering is easy. The cost is predictable. And in two minutes, they are tucked safely away into a table or car where their meal can be wolfed down. The efficient worker can be back in the office in thirty minutes or, at most, one hour.

Security in eating for the average American means there are no surprises. The majority of the fast-food outlets offer security, because the consumer knows his choice will have the same shape and taste that it had the week before.

Fast food is a repeat customer business. People return time after time to identical-sized portions. The fast-food customer values security as much as food.

Soluble Data About Fiber

It fills you up on fewer calories, reduces cholesterol, and may even combat cancer. It is no wonder that from the American Medical Association to the surgeon general to the National Cancer Institute to the American Heart Association—everybody is encouraging you to eat more fiber.

The typical American adult should consume three to four times more fiber daily, from an estimated 11 grams to somewhere between 35 and 50 grams.

According to an AMA report, dietary fiber not only helps prevent and treat constipation but also may play a role in warding off gastrointestinal disorders such as diverticulosis and perhaps heart disease. There is also some indication that a high-fiber, low-fat diet may improve control of blood sugar in diabetics and may even protect against colon cancer, although evidence on the latter is minimal.

Fiber, or "roughage" or "bulk," contributes to a feeling of satiety, assisting those trying to control calorie intake.

Most fiber passes intact through the digestive tract to the large intestine. Here some types of fiber are digested into glucose by bacterial enzymes, and the free glucose molecules are absorbed into the body. Fiber in the large intestine holds water and regulates bowel activity. Some fiber binds cholesterol and certain minerals carries them out in the feces.

Don't worry about the difference between water-soluble fiber and fiber that is insoluble. All "whole plant" foods seem to contain many types of fibers, a lot of them having both soluble and insoluble. Increase your consumption of complex carbohydrates: whole-wheat breads, whole-grain cereals, fruit, vegetables, and legumes. These foods tend to decrease consumption of foods high in fat. Look out for labels making fiber claims. There are no rules for what they can and cannot claim. It's strictly buyer beware.

Here are some foods that will help you get your recommended daily 35 to 50 grams of fiber: a small apple (with skin), small banana, two prunes, or sixteen large cherries each contribute about two grams. Cereal boxes usually indicate grams per serving, a minimum of two is recommended. One quarter cup of corn bread supplies two grams, as does 1½ cups of popped popcorn.

Two grams of fiber are supplied by ½ cup of broccoli, brussel sprouts, carrots, one large tomato or one small potato.

Half cups of garbanzo beans, kidney beans, or canned baked beans supply eight grams of fiber, as does one cup of dried peas or lima beans.

Adding purified fiber to foods, such as sprinkling bran, is not recommended. Nutritionists believe such practice can easily be taken to extremes. They also worry about taking only one isolated type of fiber, whereas fiber types in foods are mixed and usually come with a healthy component of water, minerals, and vitamins.

One important side effect to note: fiber carries water out of the body and can cause dehydration. It is very important, especially when you start to increase your fiber intake, to drink plenty of water.

There are many reasons to eat more high-fiber foods. Even if fiber does nothing more than provide regular bowel movements that's no small contribution. Americans spend $500 million annually on laxatives.

22

Poor Eating Is Bad to the Bone

If fat reduction isn't reason enough to eat sensibly and exercise regularly, I have a bone to pick. Not just one bone, but actually every one composing your skeletal system.

Mineral bone density is a precious commodity. It is abused by the likes of cigarettes, soft drinks, salt and caffeine, which cause calcium loss or block its absorption. Proper eating and effective exercise prevent or diminish chances of osteoporosis, the name given to the disease that means insidious thinning of bone tissue.

Post-menopausal, slender, small-boned, fair complexioned Caucasian women are the osteoporosis high-risk group. Synthetic estrogen helps, but there is concern about increased risk or breast, cervical and ovarian cancer.

Good eating and exercising are the cornerstones of a comprehensive plan, the fruits of which are likely never to be apparent to you. Writing in a magazine entitled *Choices*, Cherie Calbom, M.S., C.N., warns: "It's not wise to forget about the condition because we can't see the results of the good things we do to prevent it. The erosion of bone happens quietly without pain or symptom until one day there is a fracture or curvature of the spine which becomes noticeable."

There is not a cure as much as there is a method of prevention. Okay, so there is some research you haven't heard about that contends effective strength-training exercise—along with the already-established osteoporosis treatments—can restore up to 15 percent of the lost bone density. Stay tuned to the medical journals for a forthcoming report.

Meanwhile, be kind to your bones. If you think that translates merely into eating more dairy products or taking calcium supplements, be careful.

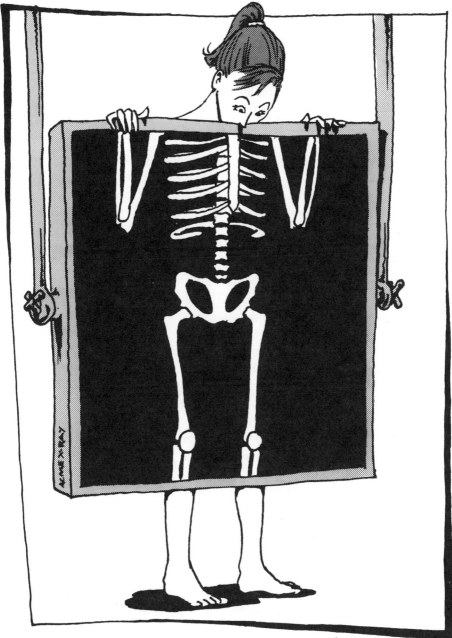

*Correct eating and exercising can diminish
your chances of osteoporosis.*

Coffee, more than two ounces of alcohol daily, and smoking all deplete calcium in the bloodstream. High-phosphate soft drinks also compete with calcium for absorption. Sugar and saturated fat adversely affect bone density, perhaps pulling calcium out of the bloodstream and into the urine.

Medical authorities can provide more scientific and detailed information. Generally, however, more calcium, magnesium, Vitamin D, boron, and anthocyanins and poranthocyanins are advisable. Where do you get these?

Calcium is the hallmark of dairy products. Be careful with accompanying fat content. Dark green vegetables such as kale, collard greens, parsley, beet greens, and broccoli are also excellent calcium sources. As for supplements, bone study contends that calcium nitrate is more effective than calcium carbonate.

Brazil nuts, tofu, dried figs, sunflower seeds, and sesame seeds also supply calcium as well as magnesium. Spinach, garlic, blackberries, whole wheat products, almonds, and cashews also supply magnesium. Sunlight is a key supplier of Vitamin D. The best food sources are sardines, salmon, tuna, shrimp, sunflower seeds, and mushrooms.

Kale, collard greens, and turnip greens provide boron, a trace mineral. Anthocyanins and proanthocyanins are pigments found in the cells of plants. They build collagen. Red grapes and blueberries are good sources.

Similar eating advice is good for preventing a great many diseases and conditions. It seems our bodies have a basic set of requirements and deviations resulting in cancers and other calamities.

As for exercise, remember that what strengthens your muscles will fortify your bones. The older, weaker, or more brittle you are, the greater the necessity of performing strength-training repetitions in a super-slow manner.

Super-slow—which means lifting the weight slowly in about ten seconds—reduces the repercussions of momentum. It's kinder and gentler to connective tissue, as well as more efficient at exercising the muscle.

This method of training, in fact, was developed by Ken Hutchins during a four-year study at the Climacteric Center at the University of Florida several years ago. Osteoporosis victims and high-risk candidates were exercised in a super-slow manner under strict supervision. Their results were astonishing.

It is not too early to start preventing hip and spine fractures that plague our elderly population. Steer your eating and exercise habits in a healthful direction.

23

Fruits and Vegetables Can Lead to Leanness

The path to thinness is lined with fruits and vegetables. Drenched in vitamins and minerals, these complex carbohydrate foods pack a nutritional wallop that can fill us up and slim us down.

The goal is to make fruits and vegetables comprise 60 percent of our daily calories. This isn't startling news. The startle comes in our failure to comply. Vague admonishments to "eat more fruits and vegetables" seem inept in the face of high-calorie gouging.

We don't like feeling denied, nor can we stand the hint of hunger. Of course, few of us really experience acute hunger. Appetite, or a craving for a particular food we find tasty, is what we often mistake for hunger. So let's not deny ourselves any particular food. Let's just assault the fruit and vegetable group.

Eat at least five servings per day. How much is that?

A serving is any of the following:

♦ One-half cup of leafy raw greens, such as lettuce or spinach.

♦ One-half cup of denser fruits or vegetables such as cauliflower, carrots, cooked spinach, or canned apricots.

♦ One-quarter cup of dried fruits such as raisins or dried apricots.

♦ A half of a grapefruit, one apple, or a medium potato.

Don't feel that you have to be a rabbit eating your way out of a garden. Five servings isn't that difficult. A cup of green beans (two servings) and a baked potato with dinner, then fruit for dessert satisfies four servings all in one meal.

Practicing vegetarians are known to enjoy better health in several aspects than comparable other people. Generally, they have lower cholesterol, fewer cases of diabetes, fewer hernias, better digestive tracts, and more desirable body weight. They suffer fewer deaths from cardiovascular disease and experience less of certain kinds of cancer.

Some of these health benefits may be attributed also to the fact that vegetarians typically abstain from alcohol and tobacco.

Vegetarian diets vary. Some include pasta, eggs and cheese, some do not. Some vegetarians eat soybean curd almost every day, and others never eat it. Some use whole foods only, relying on modern, textured vegetable protein products that are formulated to look and taste like meat, fish, or poultry.

The point here is not to convert anyone to a vegetarian eating style. That is optional. But at least five servings per day from the fruit and vegetable food group is mandatory.

At least one serving at breakfast (citrus juice), one at lunch (apple or banana), and two or more for dinner, plus a snack or two, is advisable.

Here are some other ideas for upping your fruit and vegetable intake:

♦ Keep a bowl of fresh vegetables in the refrigerator for snacking.

♦ Add lettuce and tomato on sandwiches, as well as slices of cucumber, zucchini, bean sprouts, spinach, carrot slivers, or snow peas.

♦ Toss raw or steamed vegetables into potato salad, pasta, or rice.

♦ Put grapes, apple chunks, or pineapple into coleslaw, chicken salad or tuna salad.

♦ Pack fresh or dried fruits for snacks away from home.

♦ Develop a couple of vegetarian meals to put into your regular dinner rotation.

♦ Try a frozen banana instead of ice cream or frozen yogurt.

Be careful not to contaminate your increased fruit and vegetable intake by loading on fatty toppings or dressings. This is a particular concern with baked potatoes and salads.

See how many of these suggestions you can implement immediately, or devise several of your own.

24

Get to the Meat of Food Labels

You can believe food labels to the same extent you can trust used car salesmen.

With either, deception is an art form.

Be skeptical of the bold print on food labels and even question the fine print. Wheeling your cart from one aisle to the next, know how to spot at least three of the major hazards.

♦ **#1**—A label heralding "No Cholesterol" doesn't mean it's consumption won't elevate your blood cholesterol level. Saturated fat, not actual cholesterol, is primarily responsible for low-density lipoprotein pollution of your bloodstream. Check the fine print for tropical oils: palm, palm kernel, and coconut.

♦ **#2**—If you think a "96 percent fat free" luncheon meat derives only 4 percent of its calories from fat, you've been victimized.

The label is deceptively referring to the product's weight. The numbers are more appealing when you divide a product by its weight instead of its calorie composition. There are two reasons for this.

First, fat contains nine calories per gram, compared to only four calories for grams of carbohydrate and protein. A food containing one gram of each, therefore, would provide seventeen total calories, nine of which are fat. Only one-third of its weight is fat, but 53 percent of its calories are fat.

Second, many products contain water, which contributes to weight but does not add calories.

If our mythical product above also contained one gram of water, it's fat weight would drop to 25 percent, although 53 percent of its calories are still derived from fat.

So-called 2 percent milk, for instance, derives 35 percent of its calories from fat.

To untangle this mess, multiply the products fat grams by nine and divide by its total calories. That will give you its fat composition.

♦ **#3**—There are more than a dozen names for sugar. There's sucrose, glucose, dextrose, maltose, lactose, maple syrup, corn syrup, corn sweetener, brown sugar, date sugar, raw sugar, invert sugar, honey, and turbinado sugar.

Ingredients are listed on labels in order of prominence. A product may not list a sugar in its first three ingredients, but if you add the different types together they might amount to a very sugary product.

"Sugar free," incidentally, does not necessarily mean fewer calories.

The food may contain sweeteners such as fructose or sorbitol that supply the same number of calories as sucrose, which is regular table sugar.

Being apprised of these three situations does not mean your defense arsenal is fully equipped. Look closely at all claims, particularly "fresh" and "light." Find out what they really mean.

Here are just two more and then you are on your own:

♦ **#4**—Be suspicious of oat bran or other ingredients with great marketing appeal. The product might have only a dash of oat bran and megadoses of less nutritious ingredients.

♦ **#5**—Do not think that "wheat" automatically means 100 percent whole wheat. Whole wheat should be the first ingredient listed in the fine print.

This is far from a conclusive list. The Center for Science in the Public Interest is pushing for consumer-friendly food labeling.

Until such effort bears fruit, however, approach the grocery store in the way you would a used car lot.

Help Someone Refuel Fitness Resolution

Here is a great idea for making you fit—help somebody else. Based on the premise that what goes around comes around, any help you extend will be returned to you tenfold, eventually.

Helping someone would reverse a trend. We usually tear each other down, don't we? It seems innocent and unintentional, but don't we do things like:

♦ Foist food upon others under the guise of graciousness. (Try fellowship instead of food.)

♦ Tell anybody and everybody the least bit thinner than ourselves that they don't need to lose weight. (Actually, they need to lose some and we need to lose more than some.)

♦ Poke fun at others' failed attempts to lose weight or stick to a fitness plan. (Reminding someone of past failures helps them to repeat failure.)

♦ Ridicule or even embarrass others for their success at shaping up. (Middle-aged married people who noticeably improve their appearance typically raise suspicion that they're involved in an illicit romance.)

So the first step to helping will be not to harm. But there is more we can do—learn how to be a supportive friend.

The most important thing to remember is that out of the abundance of the heart the mouth speaks—so fill your heart with tender concern for their best interest. This is the first step in adjusting our attitude.

Be it fitness or anything else, it doesn't matter how many times any of us have been knocked down. We just have to get up one more time. A helping hand makes it easier. Considering the typical life-span of new year resolutions, there have to be plenty of prospects desperate for our help right now.

If a friend or loved one has already abandoned their fitness resolution, find out what you can do to help restore it. Walk with them, talk with them, cook and freeze low-calorie meals with them—do whatever you can.

A lot of people are finding out, one-half month into a new year, that fitness pursuits test our faith. We want instant fixes and painless cures, but physical fitness does not work that way.

The first stage is always discipline. Pay the price of discipline now or the price of regret later. This discipline can be transformed into delight later as we start to see the reward for our faith and perseverance.

Do you really understand the phrase: "Fitness is a journey, not a destination"? It means that you never arrive at a point where you can permanently stop. You are forever in pursuit of either fitness or greater fitness.

Who can you help, today, in a loving way, with their fitness goals? Contact that person. Reach out to someone else. Deepen, or even develop, a friendship.

Do not underestimate the importance of this suggestion. The greatest things in life are so subtle that we often miss them.

To be a friend is to have a friend, and fit friends are even better.

26

Dining Out While Dieting

Are you perplexed about dining out and how to combat high-calorie restaurant food? Don't be, because I have some guidelines that will help you in your quest for long-term success.

Four or five years ago it was tough trying to combine dieting and dining out. Today, however, we live in a health- and fitness-conscious age. No restaurant is going to be surprised or unprepared to accommodate special requests.

This is true throughout the world. I recently spent a week in Europe and a week in Canada, eating out every meal. No matter what the cuisine—French, Italian, German, or Chinese—I managed to get what I wanted at almost every restaurant I visited.

The problem is not with the eating establishment. It's with the dieter. Some dieters just don't want to diet when dining out. Others want to but either don't know how to order or are reluctant to make demands. Here's how to deal skillfully with each situation.

The dieter who wants to cheat—You know how the story goes: You'll probably never eat here again or ever have the chance to eat these foods another time. Besides everything on the menu sounds so delicious. Maybe you're the type who can cheat just a little—overindulge only once—without running amok, but I doubt it. Most likely, a little bit of those wonderful tasting foods quickly leads to a lot.

My advice is to stick to your diet. To keep you on the right track, do not look through the menu. The purpose of the menu is to entice you to spend big, and the best restaurants really know how to sell the sizzle. Decide in advance what you want and spell it out specifically.

If you absolutely must have a high-calorie favorite, demand a half or smaller-size portion. Never order a full-size entree with the idea that you'll eat half and take the rest home for the doggie.

It's simply too tempting to consume the whole thing.

The intimidated diner—Some people feel intimidated about being assertive in a restaurant. Don't let yourself fall into this category. In most restaurants, especially the fine ones, the customer's-always-right philosophy is the rule. Restaurants are in business to satisfy customers, and most are gracious about accommodating special needs. But you have to be forthright to get what you want.

This is where most people run into trouble. Many diners are reluctant to specify anything out of the ordinary. They don't want to make waves or draw attention to themselves. Now is the time to turn your fear into positive action.

How to order—Here are the best guidelines to use when ordering your meal:

♦ Leave the menu unopened. Remember, you want to eliminate the sizzle.

♦ Ask the waiter what kind of fresh fish is available. Though chicken is as acceptable as fish, you are better off with fish, which is always prepared to order. Because of its lengthier preparation time, chicken is usually partially prepared earlier in the day with various marinades and sauces.

♦ Choose a white fish and have it baked, steamed, or broiled, with nothing on it.

♦ Inquire about vegetables and select two with nothing added. A plain baked potato is always available. Other good choices are broccoli, cauliflower, and carrots, as well as green salad.

♦ Add no croutons or bacon bits to the salad. Lemon juice and low-calorie dressing are acceptable.

♦ Request a large pitcher of ice water to be placed on your table. Drink freely before, during, and after your meal.

♦ Be assertive. Diet-conscious diners are changing restaurants by demanding a greater variety of lower-calorie foods. You'll find diet sodas, sugar and salt substitutes, caffeine-free coffee and tea, whole grain breads, fresh fruits and vegetables, and nonfat salad dressings in practically any restaurant you visit.

♦ Have caffeine-free coffee or tea for dessert, or at most, some fruit, such as strawberries or raspberries.

♦ Be very specific with your order. Double check to make sure that your waiter understands exactly what you want.

With a little practice of the above guidelines, you'll be an expert at dining out and dieting.

27

Control Your Eating Habits

Hunger is nothing to fear. Besides, rarely do we experience actual, real-life physiological hunger. Mostly we respond to cues that spur our appetite and usually result in eating binges.

"Most habitual eating is unrelated to hunger," according to James M. Ferguson, M.D., author of *Habits Not Diets*. "It is more related to the environment—the presence or reminder of food—or to an emotional state."

You might be surprised to learn what some of those cues can be: time of day, sight of food, TV commercials, friends or relatives, food aroma, a quiet house, children, your emotional state.

This list is extensive and differs with each individual.

The best way to discover what might be your binge trigger is to keep a thorough food diary: Record what you eat, in what quantity, at what time of day, in what emotional state. At least note the times you eat more than you wanted.

Then an eating plan is essential.

Know what you are going to eat each day ahead of time. Be flexible enough to change, but at least start with a plan. Don't just let eating happen!

A good supply of dietary fiber (fruits, legumes, whole grains) will help provide a feeling of fullness. Emphasize nutrient-dense foods in the range of 1000 to 1500 calories. A reduction of 500 calories a day results in a pound of fat loss in a week. It is ill-advised to skip meals. You'll only overeat later.

If these nuts-and-bolts strategies are not enough, perhaps you need to develop a bold attitude.

Welcome hunger. Aside from eating three meals and two light snacks per day, strive to be "hungry." Think in terms of: "I'm not afraid of hunger."

If you feel hungry, think of yourself becoming slim. Too many of us worry about becoming hungry or being deprived of tastes that please our palate. But nothing tastes as good as the feeling of having a strong, lean body.

28

Don't Let Dieting Consume You

It's easy to lose weight through dieting. Think of how many times you've done it. A diet is short-term deprivation featuring an emphasis on will-power. But a diet is just a 100-yard sprint in the marathon of life. No matter how many times you sprint the 100 yards, you'll never be successful at the marathon.

How about a strategy for the long haul? The most important fact about weight loss is simple: You take in calories through eating, burn them up through activity, and get fat when the calorie intake is greater than the expenditure.

You need a management system, a means of controlling the intake and maximizing the expenditure.

Are your most consistent actions the ones that promote slimness, or do they make you fat? Notice that I said "most consistent actions." You are allowed exceptions.

Here are important keys to achieving long-term success:

♦ Keep records to identify your eating triggers. A food diary is indispensable. Write down what you eat, when, and what emotions you were feeling.

♦ Review recipes and grocery lists to see whether there is a lower-calorie alternative that would be just as satisfying. Calories can be sliced from many recipes with little or no effect on taste.

♦ Abolish the all-or-nothing attitude, that of either being on or off a diet. This is the classic yo-yo syndrome. Replace this with a step-by-step plan to improve your habits, beginning with the most significant one that offers a clear-cut solution. Make changes that you can stick to for life.

♦ Maximize your incentive. Write down your goals, with definitive reasons why they are important.

♦ Replace restaurants where you typically overeat with new ones where you can make a sensible selection.

♦ Don't eat while driving the car, sitting in front of a TV, or reading a magazine or newspaper. Pay attention to the calories you are consuming.

♦ End your meals a little short of where you normally would, and get busy with something else, preferably a physical activity.

♦ Drink at least a gallon of water each day and more if you can.

♦ Take a class or launch a new hobby that does not revolve around food, or quit one that does (such as a gourmet club).

♦ Be honest about where your fitness goals rank on your priority list. If it's a low ranking, you can't expect much.

♦ Understand that you are human and that you will take three steps forward and then two steps back. This is a daily grind. Slow, steady progress brings long-term success, while instant perfection quickly shatters into thousands of little pieces.

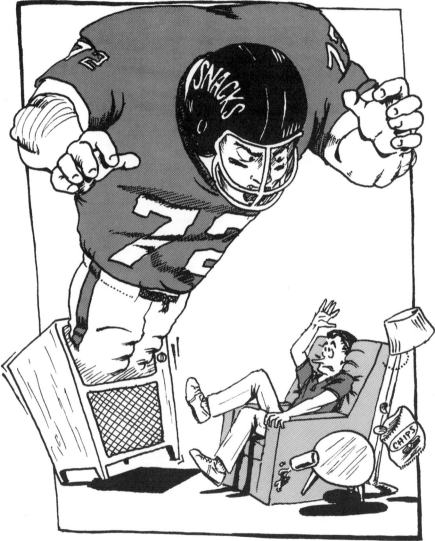

Don't let television catch you off guard.

Avoid Being Sacked by Football's Snack Attacks

If our physical pursuits in the fall of the year include playing armchair quarterback, we're sure to be sacked under an avalanche of calories.

Watching television of any sort is an invitation to overeat. Whether it's football, sitcoms, or cable news, we expose ourselves to that billion-dollar industry that excels at influencing us to enjoy the great taste of something or other. Eating is a mindless automatic reflex.

But before we're fitting into Regrigerator Perry's pants, munching our way through hours of TV football is a habit that has to change.

Here is a game plan for a lower-calorie football season.

♦ A **relish tray** (broccoli, florets, cucumbers, celery, carrots, radishes) with **non-fat yogurt** as a dip. Drink water flavored with lemon.

♦ A **fruit salad.** If slicing and dicing is too burdensome, an apple sure can fill you up and provide a great deal of oral gratification. For sweetness, put brown sugar or cinnamon on the apple.

♦ A **light popcorn** without butter. Sprinkle on Parmesan cheese for extra taste.

♦ A **high-fiber cereal** that can be eaten dry, kind of like a cookie or nuts. The best of these would be Frosted Mini Wheats.

♦ A **frozen banana** for a taste sensation almost like ice cream. **Non-fat frozen yogurt** or **ice milk** would have to be carefully rationed.

♦ Flavored **coffee** or **tea** to warm your belly. The warmth many times curbs the urge to snack.

♦ Of the popular things that come in a bag or a box and are so easy to reach into, **pretzels** are less damaging than either corn or potato chips.

That's seven points—a touchdown of good ideas. Sure, something along the lines of whole-wheat matzo crackers would be ideal, but such a level of austerity would probably cause a fumble and next week we'd be back into the nachos and nuts.

And now it's time for a field goal, three more points:

♦ No instant replays on the snacks—keep the quantity under control.

♦ Get on the floor and do some push-ups or sit-ups each time there's a score, and you won't feel like the Good Year Blimp by the time the Super Bowl arrives.

♦ If none of these strategies are moving you toward the goal line, purchase a mouth guard such as the football players use. Insert this teeth-protector as the game begins, thus putting your chompers on what the football managers term the "unable to perform" list.

Have a great season—and a healthy one!

30

Diet Saboteurs Hit Close to Home

Someone you love very much might well be standing between you and the lean physique or shapely figure of which you dream. Diet saboteurs are not highly trained foreign espionage agents—they're spouses, friends, parents, in-laws, and assorted loved ones.

Diet saboteurs identify themselves through statements such as: "C'mon, you can have just one; one isn't going to hurt you." Or: "You don't need to lose weight."

They also make high-calorie foods and beverages readily available or entice you with their self-indulgence.

These people love you, but they can't deal with the outcome they fear from your fitness goals. Diet saboteurs, you see, are comfortable with the status quo. A change in your lifestyle or appearance threatens them for several reasons.

First, they feel pressured to make a similar change. Second, they wonder if your drive to change is fueled by dissatisfaction with the relationship the two of you share. Third, they wonder what ultimately will result, particularly from your improved appearance.

Spouses and best friends sabotage instinctively and without really knowing it. Even if they give verbal support, their actions deliver a different message.

A spouse not interested in improving his or her own eating and exercising habits is bound to be annoyed by your new fitness lifestyle. You aggravate this situation if you impose a holier-than-thou attitude. Don't recite the

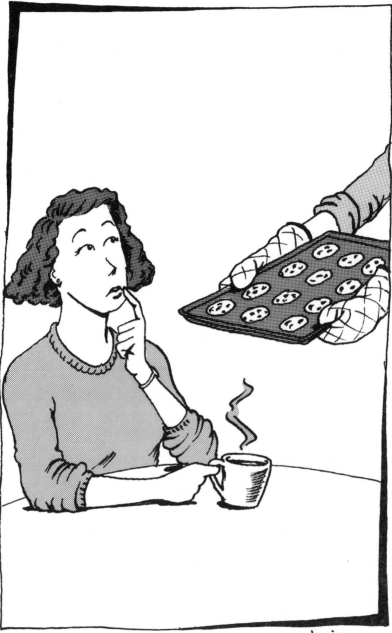

"Honey, a couple of my cookies won't hurt your diet."

calorie total in a bag of corn chips and lament the hazards of saturated fat to your mate about the quench a munchies attack.

If your mate does not share your drive for thinness, leave him or her alone. Ask for support—with plenty of explanation as to why this matter is so important. Tell this person specifically what you want them to do.

"Honey, when we go out to eat, remind me that I'm trying to fit into that black dress I want to wear to your niece's wedding next month. Make sure I order sensibly and ask for a doggie bag immediately if the portion served is too large."

Always communicate in loving, supportive terms. If hubby has made a big deal out of trying to slim down and you catch him with his hands in the peanuts watching the football game—be kind.

Compassion conquers.

The "best friend since high school" is a special species of diet saboteur. Aren't you, in a lot of ways, competing with this person? Best friends feel jealousy. Everything being relative, the thinner you become, the fatter they look.

Find a way of buttering them up. Praise them in an area apart from their fitness habits.

"I've always admired you because _____. One thing I'd really like to accomplish is being in shape. Will you help me by _____?"

Fill in the blank with a pointed, specific request. It could be something like "serving me ginger ale next time I'm at your house."

A good strategy when you're a dinner guest, incidentally, is to ask for a recipe in lieu of a second helping or a tempting dessert. This might even work with another category of saboteur—your mother.

Mothers are not trying to thwart your self-fulfillment, they're satisfying their biological need to nurture their young.

31

A Strategy for Managing the Munchies

Despite our level of dieting diligence, we all are powerless on occasion to fend off an attack of the munchies.

The times we're talking about are those for which no amount of carrots, broccoli, cauliflower, cucumbers, or fresh fruit will satisfy. Whether it's a hyperactive sweet tooth, a salt craving out of control, an ice cream avalanche, or an Easter candy catastrophe, the damage can be minimized.

Here's a strategy to put into practice.

Surround yourself with foods that provide a lot of mileage per calorie. Wear yourself out chewing. If your sweet tooth is getting the best of you, try the following:

♦ **Bread and a no-fat spread.** Whole-wheat bread—100 percent whole wheat—is highly nutritious and satisfying, weighing in a lean and mean 70 calories per slice. Serve it with jam, jelly, or fruit spread that contains zero grams of fat and you'll add approximately 35 calories of sweetness.

♦ **Apple with brown sugar and cinnamon.** Top an apple with a dash of brown sugar and cinnamon, then heat in the oven at 350 degrees for fifteen minutes. From a little apple to a big apple you'll probably range from 75 to 150 calories.

♦ **Twinkies.** A Twinkie is approximately 140 calories, but less than 30 percent fat. The typical two Twinkies per wrapper is a significant 280 calories—a lot less damage than you sustain through some of its shelf mates.

If you need something salty (and you're on a salt-restricted diet), here's a trio that conserves calories:

♦ **Orville Redenbacher's Light Natural Microwave Popping Corn.** A three-cup serving is only 100 calories, 18 percent of it fat. No-frills air-popped and a few of the hard-core diet popcorns are lower in calories and sodium, but they also taste like cardboard.

♦ **Pretzels.** Pretzels are baked, not fried, with little or no added fat. An ounce of thin pretzels instead of an ounce of potato chips will conserve forty calories and nine grams of fat. Before eating scrape off as much salt as you can manage without.

♦ **Crackers.** The low-calorie crackers are matzos, various Ry-vita crisp-breads, and Wasa Lite vintages. But don't be fooled by the words "whole wheat" or "whole grain" in the bold print on any package. Check the fine print for the ingredients.

When you're looking for something creamy, cold, and delicious, **sorbet, ice milk, Toffuti, frozen yogurt, and polydextrose products** stand ready to satisfy. Even among this esteemed group, however, calories and fat content vary. If you're really particular, therefore, check the labels (pass on the brands that do not provide nutritional information). Otherwise, just be satisfied it isn't ice cream.

Cookies that provide a little more chew-per-calorie are animal crackers and ginger snaps. Entenmann's cholesterol-free products (yellow banner on package) contain significant calories but very little dietary fat.

Once your Munchies Assault is assembled, remember that you detonate it only when you absolutely cannot hold out any longer.

Defense Is Best Offense Against Holiday Calories

The holiday season brings the office party, the family get-together, the reunion with out-of-town friends. There are the NFL playoffs and the college bowl games. Also on schedule is this or that organization's holiday bash. At the office there's a daily buffet of sweet-tooth satisfiers. A calorie consumption catastrophe is under way.

But it doesn't have to be. If you don't want to begin the new year by having your wardrobe altered a size or two larger, devise your plan of defense now.

When you're the host or hostess, serve low-calorie meals and snacks and offer more activities than just sitting and eating. Still, what happens under your own roof isn't the big problem.

You'll be eating and drinking more often at locations out of your direct control. Here are four important steps to take.

♦ **Plan ahead, eat ahead.** If the festivity includes dinner, find out what is on the menu. If there are not enough good choices, or if dinner is served well past your normal meal time, eat at home. Budget 100 to 200 calories for some polite eating at the party.

♦ **Limit alcohol intake.** It's one of the most calorie-dense foods. Alcohol also tends to be accompanied with munchies galore. As judgment blurs, there's more to drink, more munchies. Social drinking can produce a quantum leap in your daily calorie intake. Couldn't you still enjoy your party if you halved your alcohol intake?

First, never drink when you're thirsty. Quench your thirst with water. If you're having mixed drinks, drink the mixer alone every other round.

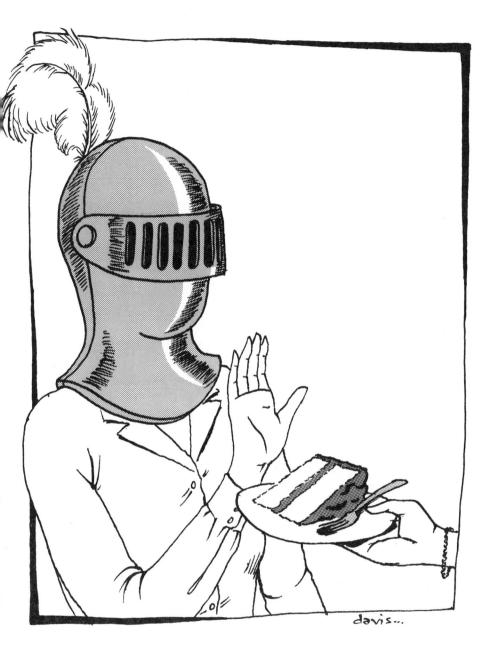

"No thank you" isn't always enough.

♦ **Say "no" firmly but gracefully.** You'll flatter the hostess—and avoid eating her mega-calorie offering—by telling her how delicious it looks and requesting the recipe. But you're unable to eat right now, darn it.

   You must be firm. This won't be easy because others will tempt you and even resent you. Tell them you have to fit into a new outfit, or give them some other specific reason.

♦ **Cut calories when not at social functions.** Trim a moderate amount from your daily breakfast, lunch, and dinner. Every meal, however, should be a well-balanced 250 calories or more. Never drop below 1,000 calories a day, unless you're under medical supervision. And never skip meals.

Call this your Calorie Consumption Catastrophe Control plan.

Concentrating on these four steps could make a difference of several pounds come the new year.

Damage Control Averts
New Year Disaster

This chapter needs a flashing red light, and maybe a siren. It needs to command your attention.

If you're buried under an avalanche of calories every January, figuring to dig yourself out from under the new year, there's still time to limit the damage. The last chapter should have started you on the right track, and here are the finishing touches.

Have you ever stopped to think how much easier it is to not gain a pound, than it is to lose one? We're talking about a legitimate pound of adipose tissue (fat), and not merely scale weight, which can be fluid and lean tissue as well as fat.

To shed one pound of fat in a week, we need to expend 500 more calories per day than we consume. To not gain a pound, we just stay even. Overeating by 500 calories each day results in an added pound after a week.

Pay now or pay later. But if you're going to put fitness on your charge account, you'll pay a greater price later.

Notions of starting a diet on January 2 is a means of absolving guilt for today's actions. Not all those who think they're going to undo the damage will muster resolve enough to see it through.

Even if you aren't only fooling yourself, cycles of on-a-diet/off-a-diet assure that you'll always be battling the bulge. Severe swings in calorie intake spell long-term disaster.

If you want some semblance of sensibility, be a smart eater while still enjoying the holidays, here are a few suggestions:

♦ Freeze some of the baked goodies you have on hand. Dole them out little by little in the coming months.

♦ If your holidays are not complete without a lot of baking and cooking, donate to those in need. A local church or charity can direct you.

♦ Cut out TV watching. Studies prove it induces needless eating.

♦ Develop daily relaxation techniques, such as deep breathing. This will take some stress out of holiday hubbub.

♦ Brush your teeth incessantly. A tingling, clean mouth won't want junk put into it.

♦ Make your slimness a Christmas present to yourself.

Body image is an emotional issue. Tame the fires of frustration right now—it will only be worse later.

Don't wait until January 2 to step on the scale to assess the damages. Intervene now.

Incidentally, hating yourself later is not the way to remove extra pounds. You've got to love being slim—not hate being fat. Concentrate on that and you won't be a helpless victim to every calorie-dense morsel within reaching distance of your tastebuds.

34

Develop a Plan to Temper Feasting

In the middle of November, when the holidays begin, you are about six weeks away from being seven pounds fatter. What a frightful thought! But it's true—the typical American unleashes a feeding frenzy through the Thanksgiving-to-New Year's season that results in an average weight gain of seven pounds.

Imagine bulging out of your favorite clothes. Think how sluggish you'll feel. Right now picture yourself with a coating of seven pounds of flab. If it's not a pretty picture, get paper and pencil and let's make a plan.

Make a statement to yourself that outlines your goals and a plan of action. The more precise, specific, and detailed, the more effective this plan will be. Start from a premise that you're going to enjoy several family feasts in the coming weeks. But to offset this calorie increase, you will decrease in other areas.

Consider incorporating the following measures, along with others you may come up with on your own.

♦ Be conscious more than ever of abundant water intake. One gallon a day will work wonders.

♦ Take 30-minute after-dinner walks on a regular basis (get up and get out quickly—you'll eat less).

♦ Read a good fitness-related book. Good means sensible, reasonable, and with claims backed by solid research.

♦ Find a nutritious vegetable soup recipe. Make a big pot and freeze in one- or two-serving plastic bags that can be thawed quickly.

♦ Cut up a relish tray (or buy one from a deli) for snacks. Use non-fat yogurt for dip.

♦ Stock up on fruit, in lieu of cookies, crackers, ice cream, and other snacks you typically buy.

♦ Perfect a couple of low-fat delicacies to take to parties. Use a magazine or cookbook that provides total calories, plus breakdowns of fat, carbohydrates, and protein. Select one less than 400 calories and less than 30 percent fat.

♦ Eliminate alcohol altogether. Besides the waistline savings, you might be avoiding DWI charges.

♦ Say no to others urging you to eat against your will. You can gracefully slide off the hook many times by asking for the recipe.

♦ Write a daily eating plan, and stick to it.

♦ Try to plan activities that are outings instead of just eatings.

♦ Select a tight-fitting New Year's Eve outfit, and try it on twice a week.

♦ Give your low-calorie home dinners the trappings of elegance—good china, candlelight, music, or whatever.

♦ Keep portions under control by incorporating nutritious low-calorie frozen dinners into your regular meal rotation. A small salad is usually needed to round out the nutrient makeup.

♦ Develop an at-home alternative workout. Coffee cans, sawed-off broomsticks, water jugs, and an assortment of other items can be used as exercise equipment.

♦ Follow up by keeping a daily journal relating to eating and exercising habits.

The gist of this action plan is that you are strict about your calorie intake whenever you're not involved in a social gathering, and you're sensible at social gatherings.

You're going to eat high-calorie foods, there's no question about it. Neither forbid nor punish yourself. To enjoy this liberty and not pile on additional pounds, however, you have to counterbalance with moderate intake at other times.

Liquid-diet shakes, incidentally, are not a good option for the strict-discipline segment of this plan. Oral gratification is needed from your food intake.

While you can pick and choose the suggestion you like, the most important thing is what not to do: Don't just cut loose; do not cast discipline to the wind. The seven-pound price you pay later will not be worth it.

35

Refining Family Recipes Pays Off

Analysis of your favorite family recipes is sure to turn up gratuitous calories. Whole milk, not skim! An entire egg instead of two egg whites! Ground beef where ground turkey or chicken would taste just the same!

Are you coming through this audit okay, or do you want an extension before we turn your recipe box inside out? This would give you time to master such things as sweating vegetables over low heat in a covered skillet, the calorie-saving alternative to frying or sautéing.

We can make a game out of this for the fun of it, and the score will eventually show around your waistline.

Research shows that the typical American family tends to eat from the same ten recipes repeatedly. The development of ten lean-as-possible recipes is a manageable task.

Challenge every ingredient, one by one. Or, you may have to rebuild from scratch—teriyaki steak kabob instead of rib-eye or turkey-beef loaf instead of meat loaf, for instance.

The specific advice here is limited by space restriction. But the magazine racks and bookstores are plump with information. Search out recipe refinements and replacements, first here and then there.

Your fondness for poultry can be enhanced by marinating a few hours before cooking. Try low-calorie salad dressings, or 1 cup low-fat yogurt, 3 tablespoons fresh lemon juice, and 1 tablespoon each minced garlic, cumin, and oregano.

Seasonings such as onion, garlic, and herbs, as well as some tomato and green pepper, will spice up ground turkey or chicken so that you won't miss ground beef.

Stir fries are a calorie-saving idea. These provide a de-emphasis on meat and poultry, with more vegetables, grains, and beans. Easy on the soy sauce.

Replace sour cream in dips and toppings with a cup of low-fat cottage cheese whirled in the blender with 1 tablespoon fresh lemon juice. Plain low-fat yogurt or buttermilk can be substituted for sour cream in salad dressings and baked goods.

Buy reduced-calorie light mayonnaise, or make your own half mayonnaise/half low-fat yogurt.

Make soups and stews a day in advance so you can chill and remove surface fat before reheating and serving.

Cut gravy calories by using arrowroot, cornstarch, or flour to thicken pan drippings. This is in lieu of roux.

For casseroles and other creamy dishes, combine 1 cup skim milk, 1 tablespoon margarine, 2 tablespoons flour, and 1/4 tablespoon salt; heat and stir until thick; then add 1/4 cup chopped celery, mushrooms, or chicken as needed. This is a low-fat, moderate-sodium substitute for condensed cream soups.

Take your low-calorie salad dressing on the side, and dip the tines of your fork into it before spearing a cluster of salad. You won't be missing any calories you could really taste anyway.

You know about non-stick skillets, or vegetable oil cooking spray preferred over pan frying, we assume? And you sauté and baste meat in broth, wine, tomato, or fruit juice instead of oil or fatty drippings?

Stock up on index cards for your recipe box. This sprinkling of suggestions and substitutions is only a start.

Gratuitous calories usually result in excess body fat.

Developing ten lean recipes based on your established family favorites is a task well worth the effort.

SECTION TWO

EXERCISING

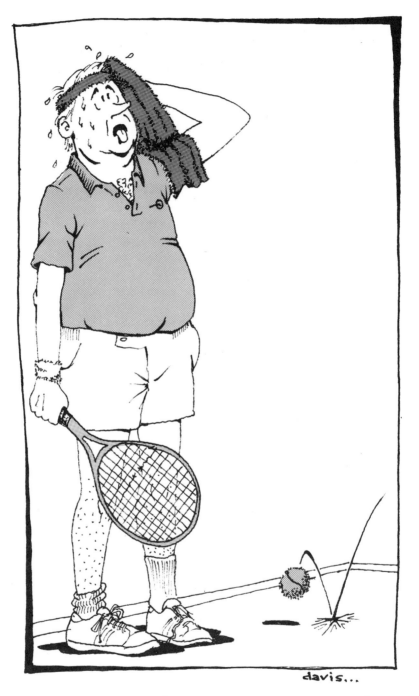

Confusing exercise and recreation is a common mistake.

36

It Isn't Exercise Just Because You Sweat

If every time you break a sweat you chalk it up to exercise, get ready for a more precise definition.

Proper exercise is a logical strategy to momentarily fatigue the major muscles of the body. Momentary fatigue appears to be the major factor required to stimulate muscular growth.

The key component of exercise is that it be demanding. These demands are manifested in labored breathing, increased pulse, elevated blood pressure, increased metabolic rate and pronounced muscle burn.

The work is so demanding that the body's physical and metabolic status quo is threatened, though not harmed. Through exercise we are sending an ultimatum to the body: "Body, your protective margins are inadequate. Adapt, enhance, improve, grow, increase . . . or you may not survive!"

Recreation should be fun. Offering vast psychological benefits, recreation is important. Play tennis, golf, softball, racquetball, basketball, and ski—they are all recreational pursuits. They should be enjoyable, while mere exercise is definitely not fun.

But recreation isn't exercise. Confusing the two can cause problems. A lot of this confusion starts at the doctor's office.

Your physician recommends that you select a leisure activity to relieve mounting stress. Exercise is also suggested but is not distinguished from recreation.

Let's say you choose to play tennis. Since tennis is rarely intense, the exercise effect is compromised.

Get into shape, then play. You should not play tennis to get into shape. You should get into shape to play tennis or any other recreational endeavor.

The reason for this is that all sports take a toll on your body. You are in danger of injury at any moment. A proper exercise program should strengthen your muscles through a full range of motion. Muscular strength provides integrity to the joints and connective tissue. It will also pack more wallop into your serve.

You need to answer three questions before undertaking a chosen form of recreation:

♦ Are you aware of the dangers involved?

♦ Are you willing to accept the dangers?

♦ Are you willing to prepare to protect yourself from these dangers?

Your choice of recreational activities is personal, but the fact that it provides pleasure and amusement is the important factor in making that choice. But please, answer the three questions posed earlier.

Exercise is demanding—and rewarding. Accept exercise for what it is—unpleasant, hard work. Do not try to enjoy it. Simply learn to endure it.

The rewards of quality exercise are increased strength, enhanced flexibility, greater endurance, better protection against injury, and improved muscle-to-fat ratio.

Some sports impart marginal exercise effect. Most of us go to a lot of trouble to have fun. Many of our chosen pastimes involve aspects of toil. But these endeavors are not exercise per se.

Physical labor, such as raking leaves or painting the garage, also provide some exercise benefit but should not be misconstrued.

Remember, exercise is a logical strategy to bring about positive physiological changes. Some changes are cosmetic, things that will be evident in your appearance. Many more relate to better health.

Too many people try to make exercise fun and, in doing so, lessen the physiological effect of the activity. Perform your exercise seriously and intensely and the quality of your life will greatly improve.

37

Take a Time-out for Exercise

It's easy to convince ourselves we're too busy to exercise. Many of us might be too disorganized to fit regular exercise into our customary routine, but the time-saving conveniences our society affords provide both the time and the reasons to pursue fitness goals.

We have the technology that makes anything more than about three half-hours of exercise each week unnecessary. Or we may use lower grades of technology for more frequent or longer duration exercise.

Use the level of technology to achieve enhanced health and greater fitness.

Here are three important components to carving time into your schedule for exercise.

♦ **Be clear about your reasons for exercising.**
What's the typical response you get from expectant parents when you ask about the desired gender? Unless there's a boy-girl imbalance in the family already, typically you hear, "I don't care, as long as he/she is healthy."

Health is the most precious quality we can wish on a newcomer to the world, and deciding to stay fit and healthy is our way of protecting that gift. There are plenty of valid and beautiful reasons for exercising regularly. Write down some of the ones that are most important to you. Reasons are leverage—they lead to solutions.

♦ **Schedule exercise time.**
We make appointments for most of our important tasks, do we not? Leaving exercise to "when I have the time," assures that we'll never get around to it. It's a cliche but true: Work expands to fill the time allotted.

Record exercise on your action list or your to do list or whatever you use for scheduling your time.

♦ **Set goals and chart progress.**
We have to know that it's worthwhile, that our devotion to exercise is leading to something. Set goals for what you want to accomplish, and then have ways of measuring your progress.

One of the best goals is to decrease resting heart rate. If you awaken leisurely in the morning (not startled by an alarm) take your pulse before getting out of bed. Write it down. Try to develop a habit of doing this every day.

Since there can be fluctuations caused by other factors in your life, take a weekly average of your waking/resting heart rate. Keep a record, chart, or graph. A couple of months later, your waking/resting heart rate should be lower.

Heart rate during exercise, and how quickly it returns to normal after exercise, are other good barometers.

A better muscle-to-fat ratio is also desirable, but this requires assessing your body-fat percentage, which you might not be able to do accurately on your own.

How many or how much of whatever exercise is yet another pertinent measurement. Log your workouts.

Devise a battery of measurements that provide meaningful feedback. Progress is motivating.

Take the time to master reasons, scheduling, goals, and progress and you'll see exercise is worth the time it requires.

Exercise Theories that Carry No Weight

People develop their own theories about exercise, based upon what they think they've experienced.

Alberta is a thirty-something female who once readily shed eighteen pounds in six weeks of a concentrated strength-training program, combined with a sensible eating regimen.

Sometime later her eating habits became unsensible and her exercise efforts ceased. She regained all the fat she had so diligently worked to eradicate.

Fed up, Alberta half-heartedly tried to re-employ the method that had worked so wonderfully before, but this time she just felt her body hardening without slimming.

Alberta, which is not the woman's real name, now believes that muscle turns to fat once you stop strength training, and when you try again to get thin, you just build muscle over fat.

If Alberta were a professional researcher, she'd have to be told that her analysis of the data is grossly incorrect. The idea that muscle turns to fat, or vice versa, is scientifically absurd.

Muscle and fat are separate tissue. One turning into the other would be like bone turning into skin, eyelashes becoming teeth, or toenails transforming themselves into warts. It just doesn't happen.

So, what is this phenomena Alberta experienced?

Muscle is very metabolically active. Its vast capillary system requires energy for blood circulation. Even at rest, each pound of muscle requires approximately 75 calories per day to sustain itself.

Therefore, when Alberta strengthened her body, she raised her resting metabolic rate. Muscle is a calorie-burning mechanism over which we can exert some influence. The nervous system also burns calories, but the only effects we can exert on it are ones that are adverse to our health and well-being.

Getting your body to burn more calories—without exertion—is a great step toward slimming down. But it works only if you can get your appetite to control calorie intake. Actually, a lot of people use exercise as a license to eat more.

Adding five pounds of muscle will raise your metabolic rate by approximately 375 calories per day, the equivalent of a candy bar. Eat two candy bars, however, and you're likely to gain fat along with muscle.

The popular term "bulking up" describes what is a combination of additional muscle and fat. While the newly built muscle could have been used to drain fat stores, the calorie overload instead increased them.

Fat, incidentally, has a metabolic load, too. Each pound of fat requires two calories per day. If you lose five pounds of fat, therefore, your resting metabolic rate drops by 10 calories per day.

But, if you quit strength training and five pounds of muscle atrophies, your metabolic rate drops by 375 calories.

Without a corresponding decrease in calorie intake, you'll get fat. And when most people stop exercising, they usually increase rather than decrease calories.

When Alberta started exercising again, her expectations were that it would be easy. Every time you lose and regain fat, however, it becomes tougher to get rid of it the next time.

Alberta remembered the conclusion of her previous experience and not the beginning of it. She remembered the fat rolling off but not the diligence she exerted over her eating habits.

Now she has some grossly mistaken concepts of proper exercise.

Strength training—hard, brief workouts on non-consecutive days—is a more efficient use of your time than aerobic-based programs.

Added muscle burns calories—added muscle that is being sustained while you sit at your computer, drive the car, or lounge on the couch. Sure you could jog, swim, or go to a dance class six times per week and use only exertion to burn the same number of calories, but you'd have to devote five hours a week to exercise instead of the 60 to 90 minutes that's needed for effective strength training.

Don't fall for the notion that to lose fat you have to exercise aerobically. This is yet another incorrect analysis of data and one that is common even among seemingly qualified exercise professionals.

The type of fuel used during exercise is not a factor in fat loss. The fuel burned during energy production is replaced during and after the exercise by foods eaten, stored carbohydrates and stored fats.

The hazard with Alberta is that believing as she does, she'll rely on a less-efficient exercise method and skirt the issue of controlling her calorie intake.

Fitness Means Action, Not Excuses

In his book, *Getting Physical: How to Stick With Your Exercise Program,* Art Turock poses three thought-provoking questions:

1. Do you want to go through life being self-conscious about your weight?
2. Do you want to go through life feeling fatigued at day's end, having to decline appealing evening opportunities?
3. Do you want to go through life putting your body at greater risk of disease and even shortening your life span?

Writing in a fitness industry publication, Turock contends, "Although most individuals would answer NO to these questions, inactive people's actions say yes."

Less than one in five adult Americans exercise on a regular basis. A whopping 59 percent are pure-bred couch potatoes, according to the National Sporting Goods Association.

For those struggling to make exercise a lifetime habit, here are some points to ponder:

♦ Expect exercise to be rewarding, not fun. Exercise is a formula designed to bring about positive physiological changes. You can have fun being in shape through recreational activities, but these are not exercise, despite some degree of exercise benefit. The process of getting yourself into shape should be strictly business.

♦ Hire a qualified trainer or recruit an exercise partner. Surveys clearly show that you stand a better chance of sticking to a program if you're not in it alone. A trainer can help you achieve results efficiently, but even your spouse commiserating through workouts with you will add incentive.

♦ Generate your motivation immediately. You're going to have cycles of ups and downs. Exercise hard during down cycles, and harder during up cycles. Do not wait for a wave of motivation. You don't have to feel like exercising, just do it.

♦ Regular exercise carves out its own time. Increased alertness and productivity should make time spent exercising time well spent. It is an investment. Do not try to flatter your feeling of self-importance by claiming that you don't have the time.

♦ Set a regular schedule and stick to it. No excuses! Attach your exercise time to another commitment. Just before or immediately after work, perhaps, or right after you drop the kids off at school or just before you pick them up. Make it an extension of another commitment.

♦ Set realistic goals that target long-term, long-lasting results. Fitness is a journey, not a destination. It should not be treated as a quick fix or a seasonal project. It should be factored into your weekly routine, the same as any hygiene.

♦ Remember that exercising slows aging. There's no question about it. The well-conditioned sixty-year-old is the equivalent of a sedentary forty-year-old.

Join the elite group—the 17 percent of adult Americans who reap the benefits of regular exercise. Join now and enrich your life immediately. Answer those first three questions with action!

40

Put More Muscle in Your Workouts

This may not occur regularly, or even very often. But sometime in the future you'll face a remodeling project, a landscaping task or be forced to move your furniture. Whatever the call to action, you'll want all the muscle you can muster.

Muscles perform work. They are the engines of the cables attached to the levers (bones) in our bodies that produce movement. Their working condition also provides a measure of protection against injury.

If you're recruiting helpers, you may want to match genetic makeup to the project at hand. This is important because there is enduring strength and explosive strength and all the points in between. What this means is that physical strength is measured as an amount of force over a period of time. We are all physiologically designed to excel at different tasks.

Some people are good at carrying ten-pound boards all day long. That's enduring strength (a little bit of force over a long time). Others are useful for lifting a fifty-pound deck into position several feet above ground. That's explosive strength (a lot of force in a little bit of time). Our suitability for a specific strength is determined genetically. The same basic formula of strength development works equally well for about two-thirds of us. Others need higher or lower dosages of repetitions and sets.

Any type of physical project can illustrate why a fitness program should emphasize muscle development and not aerobics. Short-rest circuit strength training, in fact, is an effective blend of both anaerobic and aerobic training.

Perhaps if a stair-climbing machine could be hooked up to a generator to run some power tools, then those people who readily overemphasize such devices might put their training to use. In real life, however, a stair-climbing machine is good only for making you better at using a stair-climbing machine. Aerobic training can be used to supplement a strength-training program, but too many people do just the reverse—a little bit of strength training and a lot of aerobics. The user-friendliness of electronic devices is one of the reasons for this, another is the dynamic instruction in an aerobics class.

Good strength training beats even the best in aerobics every time. You'll notice this next time you spend several hours lifting, standing, painting, raking, mowing, or hanging wallpaper. Good muscular condition will make you more productive and help to withstand aches and pains (although lots of projects overstress a particular joint such as the hand or elbow).

You might even avoid the day-after backache. It's easy to understand this when you recognize how the spine functions.

The vertebrae, along with the muscles and tissue that connect them, provide the framework that keeps us upright. They are also conduit for the spinal cord, which is an extension of the brain and a freeway of nerve impulses, hormones, and chemicals.

If any of the bones that protect the spinal cord happen to slip or twist out of line, the size or shape of the opening where the nerve trunk comes through can change. This is a condition known as vertebral subluxation.

The paravertebrals—the muscles which run parallel to the spine—

function like cables to provide stability for the vertebrae, which are stacked with discs in between. These muscles also flex and extend (bend and arch) the spine. The greater the strength of the paravertebrals, the better the spinal protection.

Any type of abnormal activity, however, may throw your spine out of alignment.

Chronic muscular contraction and tension can also alter the normal nerve supply. When this happens, the organs, glands, and tissues that depend upon the nerve supply may suffer. Impaired nerve force often causes pain, loss of function, and even disease.

Stronger muscles can help you avoid discomfort. You'll find this out the next time you tackle a demanding project.

41

Slower Strength Training Speeds Muscle Building

One of the most popular forms of exercise today is strength training. It usually involves the lifting and lowering of weights in the form of barbells, dumbbells, or various exercise machines.

The majority of people involved in strength training perform their repetitions too fast. They need to slow down. Doing so is safer and more productive.

Using the type of training I'm about to describe resulted in fifteen pounds of additional muscle onto an already muscular young man who trained for just six weeks one summer in Dallas. The first diet group (one made up of ninety women) to employ this type of exercise produced 59 percent better results than earlier groups who trained more traditionally.

This new style of exercise is called super-slow training, and it was developed principally by Ken Hutchins of Orlando, Florida. What super-slow means is ten seconds to lift the resistance, turn around smoothly at the top, lower in five seconds, smoothly turn around at the bottom and lift again in ten seconds. That's ten seconds up, five seconds down, with smooth turnarounds at each end.

Super-slow is a much harder, more intense training. You have to cut back the resistance you use by about 40 percent.

Slow repetitions rely more on muscular contraction and less on momentum. Conversely, the faster the repetition the more momentum you've recruited—and the less muscle you're using.

A high-velocity repetition involves a great thrust at the initial point of movement. Over the last half of the range of motion, however, momentum carries most of the load. The muscles are not being taxed.

In exercise we're not looking to make it easier, we're looking to make it effective.

Metabolic work—primarily what your muscles are doing—is far more important than the action of the weight whose movement is mechanical work.

Fast, jerky repetitions also do not effectively isolate individual muscle groups, and proper isolation is important in complete muscle strengthening. Furthermore, fast repetitions generate an impact that reverberates in your joints and connective tissues.

Move slower, never faster, if in doubt about the speed of movement on each repetition. This is one of the basic principles of strength building. Yet it is one of the first that is violated by most trainees. It is violated because it is easier to move fast and jerkily than it is to move slowly and smoothly. Ten-second lifting repetitions soon become a painful, fatiguing experience.

Decide now that you want to get the best-possible results from your strength-training program. Slow down.

42

Making a Stronger Case for Building Muscle

In his search for the fountain of youth, Ponce de Leon would have been better off at Muscle Beach.

Concerning the so-called normative changes associated with aging, William Evans, Ph.D., of the USDA Human Nutrition Research Center was recently quoted as saying, "It's changes in muscle mass that may be triggering all of the other changes."

Evans was addressing a meeting of the American Dietetic Association, as reported in the May/June 1990 issue of *Food Insight*. He cited research in which forty-five- to sixty-year-old athletes were compared to athletes age twenty-something, as well as inactive men in both age groups. Researchers found that the loss of muscle and increased fat were not age related.

"We can see that the amount of fat they have stored is directly related to the amount of time they spend exercising," says Evans.

Evans also referred to research in which eighty- and ninety-year-olds increased the size and strength of their leg muscles. At the ADA meeting, he seemed to be lending his voice to the chorus of experts telling us that creeping obesity is making us old before our time.

Our muscle mass, principally, can keep us younger longer.

There is another study that possibly not even Evans has paid much attention to. It was published in 1975 by a research group headed by Dr. Alfred L. Goldberg.

In working with laboratory rats, Goldberg found that if muscle is stimulated to grow through exercise, it will grow in defiance of tremendous adversity and at the expense of the remainder of the organism.

Why?

One of the fundamental traits of animal life is locomotion. Locomotion depends on muscular size and strength. Survival resources are, therefore, allocated to the muscles first. This priority allocation depends on muscular growth stimulation.

When we stimulate our muscles to grow, they pull energy (calories) from our fat stores.

Muscles have a vast capillary system and, other than nerves, are the biggest energy user in the body. This is why every pound of muscle we can grow raises our metabolic rate by approximately 75 calories each day.

If we do not use our muscles significantly they will atrophy. Instead of increasing metabolic rate, the rate will decrease. This is what typically happens as we get older; we lose muscle through inactivity. Simultaneously, we increase our caloric intake.

A slight but consistent reduction in calorie intake, coupled with an increase (or at least not a decrease) in muscle mass keeps our waistlines in check and our energy high.

Perhaps it also bolsters our immune system. Perhaps more fruits and vegetables and fewer deep-fat-fried foods and hydrogenated oils restrict the chances of malignant growths or clogged arteries.

Perhaps the heavy breathing induced by exercise cleanses our lymph system.

Perhaps if we realized that benefits accrue over extended periods of time, we wouldn't lose our patience and junk our resolve.

Perhaps youth and vitality do not have to fade from our grasp so quickly.

We can strongly influence this situation—there's no perhaps about it.

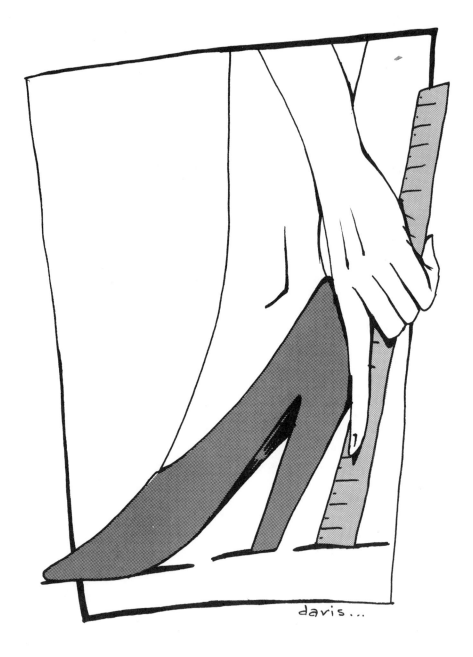

When you wear over three-inch heels do your feet hurt?
If so, try the one-legged heel raise.

43

The Lowdown on Heels

High heels add sway to your hips, length to your legs, and shape to your calves. They can help you look taller, more elegant, more professional, and even sexier.

In two-to-three inch heels not only do your buttocks protrude more, but, in doing so, you must arch your spine and pull your shoulders back to keep from falling on your face. This has an uplifting effect on your breasts. Protruding buttocks and uplifted breasts usually connote sexual attractiveness.

Wearing high heels, however, can also cause problems. According to a recent Gallup poll, more than half of the women that wear high-heeled shoes complain that their feet and ankles hurt. Much of the pain is caused by a tightening of the Achilles tendons, the link between the calf muscles and the heel bones.

When you stand flat-footed, these tendons are stretched. In high heels, they are bunched up and contracted. Wear high heels long enough, and this can turn into a problematic condition. So what's the solution—give up high heels altogether?

Even podiatrists know that is unrealistic. High heels are too much a part of our culture.

The solution is moderation and a simple exercise.

Try to change back and forth between high heels and flats. Also, experiment with a pair of medium-heeled shoes.

For a simple exercise to stretch and strengthen your Achilles tendons, I recommend the following movement before you go to bed at least three nights a week. Furthermore, this exercise will add shape and contour to your calves.

One-legged heel raise: Wear flat, rubber-soled shoes. Stand on a sturdy step or ledge that is at least four inches high. Balance your body weight on the ball of your left foot only. Hold onto a railing or wall for support.

Raise your left heel slowly and try to stand on your big toe. Pause. Do not bend your knee. Keep it straight throughout the movement. Lower your heel smoothly until it is well below the step. Stretch. Repeat the slow, smooth raising and lowering of your left heel for ten repetitions.

Follow the same procedures with the right foot.

Since the range of movement on the heel raise is so short, it's best to work up to twenty repetitions with each leg.

Practice the one-legged heel raise three times per week for a month and you'll increase significantly the strength and flexibility of your lower legs.

44

Stand Muscle Pain to Get the Gain

One of the big limitations that shackles people from achieving results from their fitness program is an intolerance to muscle-burn pain.

If you've ever been on a Nautilus machine or attempted a heavy bench press, you know the sensation. It's a rush of lactic acid caused by an oxygen debt in the muscle.

For whatever reason, this sensation is most evident in the frontal thigh, the quadriceps muscle. This is where the vast majority of people seem to be the most sensitive. But the calves, shoulders, and upper arms also induce their share of muscle burn.

You've got to be able to stand the pain if you want the results.

These painful reps are the ones that make the difference. Those that preceded them were just a warm-up. If you stop short of a good burn you've just spun your wheels—and you're not progressing.

You have to distinguish beneficial muscle-burn pain from the harmful pain of muscle strain or connective tissue tears. This isn't difficult. Focus on the burning sensation, as opposed to the tearing sensation.

Oxygen is the key player in exercise.

Anaerobic exercise is that which is carried to the point of fatigue of the specific muscle targeted by the exercise. This is commonly referred to as strength training or weight lifting.

Aerobic exercises are those in which oxygen is continuously pumped into all the working muscles. The fatigue that is ultimately encountered is that of the pumping system and not an individual muscle or group of muscles.

Exercise physiologists tend to lump exercises into all-or-nothing columns—either it's aerobic or anaerobic.

A marathon run is truly an aerobic endeavor. A one-repetition-maximum barbell dead lift is truly an anaerobic experience. But these are extremes.

Most of the exercises you and I do are blends of aerobic and anaerobic. The richest blend of these is circuit strength training performed with no wasted motion in getting from one exercise to the next. It's the most time-efficient overall exercise program in existence.

In a properly orchestrated circuit of strength-training exercises, the cardiorespiratory system is continuously taxed to near capacity.

While this is going on, anaerobic thresholds are encountered systematically from one muscle group to the next throughout the entire body.

The rigors of this process are very beneficial.

Straining for oxygen during strenuous exercise produces a respiratory rate increase of three to five times its resting rate. Air is pulled into the lungs when you inhale, putting oxygen into the bloodstream.

Breathe freely during exercise. Short, shallow breaths—kind of like a dog panting—work best.

Triggering this type of heavy breathing through exercise on a regular basis is a great health enhancement. Toxins are released. Some contend also that the lymph system is cleansed.

How much muscle burn can you stand? The muscle fibers are not being ignited, as you may feel. It's just this chemical process going on. Challenge it to the max.

If your doctor could write you a prescription that would control your blood sugar, lower your blood cholesterol, lower your blood pressure, help you lose weight, and increase your energy level, would you take it?

Then start exercising from today and on through forever.

45

Reap Rewards of Unfun Exercise

Of all the misguided information concerning exercise, the most frustrating is the notion that it should be fun. The reasoning goes, "Whatever exercise you do should be fun, or you won't stick with it."

I'd like a nickel for every time the past several weeks I've heard or read such a statement—and some antacid tablets to soothe the resulting sick feeling in my stomach.

Have fun and you're sure to stay unfit. As I've stated previously, exercise should be rewarding, not fun. It should bring about physiological change, not psychological amusement. Fun is the antithesis of exercise.

The reason that we exercise is to get our body to change, is it not? Fun workouts are such because the demands we place on our bodies remain within the limits of our existing capabilities. That doesn't work.

We have to nudge beyond our limits to force our bodies to adapt to an increased demand. Very few of us consider muscle burn, fatigue, and nausea—the by-products of effective exercise—to be fun. Yet these are the requirements if we are to benefit from a fitness program.

If you accept a broad definition of exercise, such that any type of exertion fits under its umbrella, your fitness level is sure to suffer. May we suggest something useful?

Consider exercise to be a strategy, meaning it is a course of action designed for a specific purpose. The purpose is to bring about an improvement in our physiology.

Exercise is a strategy enacted to produce physiological improvement. Let's tell Webster!

Fun is wearing a size of clothing we haven't fit into in years. Fun is having people complement our appearance. Fun is performing a task that was previously difficult and now having it seem easy due to our enhanced fitness level.

Fun is the fruit of the endeavor itself.

There is another qualification of proper exercise—it should be brief. Whenever anyone brags about how much they work out, you can be sure they're not in very good shape.

I've mentioned Arthur Jones's quote that "there is no such thing as a long, hard workout" before. The terms contradict each other. A workout that is hard has to be brief. And if it is long, it couldn't have been that hard.

There are a lot of people who have brief moments of hard workouts amidst a lot of wasted time between exercises. Their workouts are effective, just not efficient.

Maybe it's fun to strut to the water fountain and look into the mirror to see your biceps bulging, but the arm curls that produced the bulge weren't very much fun.

On a 10-exercise circuit of intense strength training if you can do eleven exercises, you didn't do the first ten hard enough. You should get from one exercise to the next quickly. If you can talk easily you're probably not giving your best effort.

On aerobic exercises, you'd better work up to a level that requires you to breathe like a freight train and stay at that level until just before you feel ready to pass out.

Genuine exercise is ugly, there is no question about it. It isn't fun, it's rewarding.

If you think this is merely a semantics peccadillo, tell me—is childbirth fun? Is getting up in the middle of the night with a sick infant fun? What if you read articles that said "child rearing has to be fun, or you won't stick with it"?

Most of the articles incorporate the fun disclaimer when trying to guide your selection of exercise method. What type of exercise is right for you? Probably the one you hate most. You hate it because it is forcing your unwilling body to change.

Do you want to exercise to amuse yourself, or do you want to produce change—and then go have some fun?

46

It Takes More than Just Muscle

Every fitness club has at least one, if not several. You've noticed him, or maybe it's a woman. But males are more sensitive to this situation and, hence, usually this person is male.

The guy we're talking about is the one for whom almost the entire weight stack is possible on most Nautilus machines. And the perplexing thing is that this individual's physique would make him a target for sand in his face at the beach. From where does his strength come?

Muscle mass is not the only factor involved in generating movement, or what we'll call strength output.

Neurological ability and bodily leverage (involving attachment points and angles of insertion of tendons into bone) increase or decrease measurable strength.

You see, a muscle does only one thing—it produces force. That force is then routed through a filtration system before movement occurs. You may have noticed that almost all champion weightlifters lack the muscular size of advanced bodybuilders, yet they are much stronger.

You may also have noticed that many men with outstanding degrees of muscular size are not very strong, certainly not as strong as they look. This phenomenon is explained by a statement from a four-time world power-lifting champion named John Kuc.

"The bones and joints form a system of levers in the human body with the muscular system providing force and movement to the levers," Kuc says. "The force that a joint can exert by flexion or extension is determined by the point of muscle insertion into the bone. Heredity has complete control over this. This accounts for two people of equal musculature and body weight having different strength levels."

Besides attachment points and angles of insertion, bone length is also a factor. A bone plays the role of a lever, so its length dictates the necessary inch-pounds of work.

Those with a body-builder's physique may have poor leverage. A great mass of muscle would be required to lift only an average amount of weight. That may be part of the reason that the muscles of body-builders grow so large.

A champion weightlifter, on the other hand, benefits from exceptional leverage. This person may not need much muscle force to lift a heavy weight.

Neurological ability is a separate factor altogether. But neurological ability makes a big difference.

A man with only an average amount of muscular bulk, but having a superior nervous system, will produce more strength output than an individual having superior muscle mass but not the ability to contract a high degree of it all at once.

Length of bone, length of muscle attachment points, and neurological ability are genetically determined. There is nothing you can do to change them. But proper strength training will maximize your genetic potential. Just be careful whose face you kick sand into.

47

The Key to Maximizing Exercise

What is Greg Norman's demeanor when he's about to tee off, or Monica Seles's when she's preparing to serve? Is Michael Jordan joking with his teammates when he's eyeing a free throw?

All of these athletes are in deep states of concentration. They're probably even visualizing the successful execution of their respective feats. Norman's golf scores, Seles's tennis ranking, and Jordan's point-per-game average would all suffer immensely if they did not put their minds into it.

Now, walk into any fitness center and what you're likely to witness is an adult romper room. Jokes, small talk, goofing-off proliferate.

Many, in fact, try to take their minds off their physical endeavor. What would Norman, Seles, and Jordan be if they did the same?

Your exercise benefits are adversely affected by a lack of concentration. You're hampering the physiological results you could otherwise be receiving.

To get the best workout you possibly can, you must concentrate. You must put your mind into it, not take it off of it.

Bob Sikora, who has trained many professional athletes and is currently a one-on-one strength trainer in Ohio, allows no small talk during any of his exercise sessions.

"I don't want to hear anything except what they're feeling from the movement," explains Sikora. "It's all business."

Ken Hutchins, a Nautilus training authority, has coined a concept he calls internalization.

"Pretend that you're in a darkened room," writes Hutchins. "No sound—other than your own bodily functions—is heard. Your only communication sense with your body is feel. In the dark, you must imagine your body parts and what they are doing. This imagery is the basis for proficient motor control. It is also the foundation for superior mental control. It is required to perform intense muscular contraction."

Mental prowess is important. Going through the motions of an exercise means very little.

True exercise should be defined as logical strategy to bring about positive physiological change. Your body's desire to maintain status quo makes producing change a very demanding experience.

True exercise is rewarding. An activity that produces fun should be classified as recreation, with perhaps a small dose of exercise effect.

If you're not convinced to concentrate but have to share workout facilities with those still having fun, maybe you should practice a task used by Russian athletes.

Get two radio or tape players and tune them into two different talk programs. Put each at the same volume. Now concentrate on just one, and in your mind tune out the other one.

Try this routine for five minutes a day for the next week. Once you get skilled at it, your exercise results are sure to improve.

Muscle Into the
Newest Fashions

A fashionably dressed woman this year will be exposing a good portion of her upper-to-middle back region, from the neck down past her shoulder blades. She will need a proud set of shoulders to present a V-shaped torso, reproportioning her figure to make her waist and hips look smaller.

Designer fashions will require a little of your own material, in addition to the mastery of Liz Claiborne and others. Muscular development, especially in the back and shoulders, is an accessory that only you can provide.

Think in terms of spot production, which means producing figure-shaping muscles in a specified area.

Most women are capable of such production, in contrast to the impossibility of spot reduction—the loss of specific fat. Exercise cannot pinpoint fat stores to be eradicated, but it can make targeted muscles bigger, stronger, more attractive to look at, and firmer to the touch. Even if there is fat in the area, muscle will help to hold it in place instead of just letting it sag.

A weak back tends to feature protruding shoulder blades and overall narrowness. This accentuates the waist, hips, and buttocks, where a woman generally stores a large percentage of her body fat.

Strengthened back muscles fan out the entire torso and set the shoulder blades flat into the back surface. There might even be some muscle definition apparent, since little fat is generally stored in this region.

A strong back also feels firm, whereas a weak one feels like loose skin resting atop a pile of bones.

If you think broad shoulders are a phenomenon of the male physique only, check your dresses, jackets, and even T-shirts. Women's fashions today have more padding in the shoulder sections of each of those garments than Joe Montana wears on Super Bowl Sunday.

Shoulder pads were first popularized in the 1940s by actress Joan Crawford. Decades later the fashion designers of the TV show "Dynasty" desired a similarly powerful, intimidating look in the Alexis character played by Joan Collins.

It's claimed that shoulder pads give a woman a forceful physical presence, along with helping to make an hour-glass figure. They mask bad posture and sloping, inadequate shoulders. Furthermore, says one fashion authority, "They make even cheap dresses hang right."

Your own muscular shoulders will save embarrassment when wearing shoulderless clothing and keep padded clothing from appearing to be hollow underneath.

So, how do you spot-produce muscle into your shoulders and back? Your figure for the nineties will require strengthening of the rhomboids and latissimus dorsi (upper and middle back muscles), along with the deltoids (shoulder muscles).

All of these muscles move the arms, specifically the upper arms. The back muscles perform all pulling motions with the arms in front of the torso. The deltoids, chief muscles of the shoulder socket, raise the arms in any direction.

A qualified exercise instructor will be able to set up an effective strength-training program for you. Just be sure to perform all your exercises slowly and smoothly.

Once you pack solid muscle into your shoulders and back your friends will admire the firmness and fitness you display. They will also marvel at how well you flatter the latest designer fashions, optimizing your attractiveness.

49

Muscle Out Extra Fat by Weight Training

A ndre Agassi's rise to the upper echelon of professional tennis, TV commentators contend, is due in part to a strengthening program that packed fifteen pounds of muscle onto his physique.

In the days of Rosewall, Laver, and Ashe—not that long ago—a tennis player would just as likely play without strings in his racket as he would build muscle mass. They mistakenly equated bulk up with slow down.

Even if you're not a mega-dollar professional athlete, physical strength is important in your life.

Okay, so how strong do you have to be to sit at a desk during the day and lounge on a couch at night? You can flip the switch on the computer, dial a cellular telephone, operate a TV/VCR remote control, punch the dials on a microwave, pull the tab on a soft drink can, and be patient enough to wait for elevators.

What use are bulging biceps in the society of the micro chip?

The machines made by man can't replace the machine that is man.

Muscles are the engine of the body; they perform work. Arthur Jones, inventor of Nautilus, told us so a couple of decades ago. And it's true.

Muscles get Andre Agassi from the baseline to the net, and they either pack more power into his strokes or provide a greater number of powerful strokes before tiring.

Muscles are where energy is released, power is produced, and where movement originates. Because the condition of our engine has a lot to do with the way we look, feel, and function, strong muscles are very advantageous.

As the engines of the body, our muscles burn fuel (calories). It's estimated that each pound of muscle requires approximately seventy-five calories for sustenance at rest (basal metabolic rate).

If you're not putting forth a serious effort in the weight room at least a couple of times per week, you're forfeiting about one half pound of muscle per year. That's how much will atrophy. This lowers your metabolic rate. If there is no corresponding reduction in caloric intake, the result is a gain of body fat.

Excess fat is unhealthy—and, to most people, unappealing.

The body's shape is determined by bone structure and muscle-to-fat ratio. More muscle and less fat improves most people's physiques. Within genetic parameters (about which you can do nothing), muscle adds shape and firmness to the body.

Strength training is the only exercise that simultaneously increases muscle and decreases fat.

If you think you have to burn body fat aerobically, you're wrong. The immediate energy source is irrelevant. You'll break down fat stores in your body to replace muscle glycogen that was burned during anaerobic exercise (strength training). Increased muscle will need more fuel from fat stores.

In addition to being the engine of the body, muscle is also the shock absorber. Strength enhances the integrity of the joints, guarding against painful tears in the connective tissues of the knees, neck, shoulder, elbows, ankles and—above all—the lower back.

More and more elements of our society are awakening to strength training's benefits: improved physical capacity, increased metabolic rate, reduced risk of injury, and enhanced physical appearance. Make sure you do, too.

50

The Age-Old Weight Control Remedy

Are you aware of your fat-gaining danger zone? Between what ages do you think you're most likely to have a girth spurt?

The Centers for Disease Control recently reweighed almost 10,000 men and women whose weight had been recorded ten years earlier in a separate study. These people ranged in age from twenty-five to seventy-four when they first weighed.

They found the following statistics:

♦ Women of all ages were twice as likely as men to experience a weight gain of 20 percent or more.

♦ Women between the ages of twenty-five and thirty-four who were overweight ten years ago had the highest chance of posting a major weight gain.

♦ For men and women of normal weight when first measured, ages thirty-five to forty-four were the fattest. Sixteen percent of the men and 14 percent of the women became overweight during those years.

We get fatter as we get older, you'll be startled to know. The typical fifty-five-year-old man and woman each notices the scale about thirty pounds above where it had been some thirty years earlier.

Furthermore, the scale isn't quite so obvious to point out that a half-pound of muscle per year dwindles away through lack of use. This means another fifteen pounds of fat, hidden from the scale but obvious in our clothes and to our health. We can't do anything about getting older. But weight is within our realm of control.

A group concerned with firefighters suggested on a recent TV program that weight gain—and not age itself—is responsible for most of the decline in performance after age forty.

"Maintaining appropriate body composition can improve performance in over-forty age group by as much as thirty percent," said one of the program's guests.

Non-smoking firefighters who keep themselves physically fit are "physiologically similar to people up to twenty years younger," this expert also said.

If you're looking for the fountain of youth, cast away your cigarettes, cut down on saturated fat intake, and elevate exercise to the status of hygiene habit.

Most people are going to get into shape someday, or so they tell themselves. It's in the plan for the future—that nebulous, distant point that never quite seems to arrive.

These people concede the benefits that are to be gained. They acknowledge the necessity of fitness in their lives.

But they never quite reach the point where they take action. There's never a shortage of excuses.

Even a high percentage of first-time heart attack victims excuse themselves from a fitness lifestyle. But this percentage drops dramatically after the second heart attack.

If we're not addressing healthful habits, then we're certainly on the fat track. Some intervention is necessary.

God forbid it should take two heart attacks to prompt action.

51

Here's How to Master Efficient Exercise

To get into really good shape, on three nonconsecutive days this week you need to do the following:

Perform one set each of at least six strength-building exercises. Maximum number of exercises is twelve. The duration of each exercise should be one to two minutes of continuous muscular tension, meaning don't relax, not even for an instant.

The repetitions should be performed slowly and smoothly. How slow? As slow as you can without there being stops or snags along the way. Ideally, this means about ten seconds to bring the targeted muscle from its full stretch to full contraction. Then, release and lower the weight in about five seconds. Slowly and smoothly start the next repetition. Do not set the weight down.

Keep performing repetitions until fifteen seconds of immovability. This means that you're trying to lift the weight, but you can't move it. Ideally, the selected resistance (weight) should cause this to happen somewhere between one and two minutes. Depending on how slowly you're performing the repetitions, this could mean anywhere from two to twenty. The slower you move, the fewer the repetitions.

At the conclusion of each exercise, move rapidly to the next. The next machine should be set for you. If your breathing is labored to the point where you cannot talk, rest a little. But if you can talk, you should be performing the next exercise.

The sequence of exercises should start with the larger muscles and progress to the smaller ones. This means from buttocks, to thighs, to upper back, to chest, to shoulders, to arms, to stomach.

Your circuit of strengthening exercises should require between fifteen and thirty minutes. You'll know if the exercises are effective by the level of fatigue after each one. On leg exercises, for instance, you shouldn't be able to get off the machine and immediately walk normally. If you can walk and look sober, either perform more repetitions or increase the weight.

You should be breathing heavily, and your heart rate should be elevated during the course of these exercises. Do not rest. Beating your body into fatigue is the name of this game. That's the only way it will change to respond to the load you place on it.

Muscle mass burns calories—that's why we work to build, or at least maintain, strength. A recent study compared those who exercise aerobically for thirty minutes to those who strength train for fifteen minutes and then exercised aerobically for fifteen minutes. Eating and all other factors in the study were identical.

The aerobics-only group lost three pounds of fat and one-half pound of muscle in eight weeks. The group that did fifteen minutes of strength training and fifteen minutes of aerobic conditioning lost ten pounds of fat and gained two pounds of calorie-burning muscle.

Don't put up with supposed experts who recommend only aerobic exercise for fat loss. In fact, if you can do only one or the other, strength train.

But be sure to do at least six strengthening exercises in approximately fifteen minutes. For another fifteen minutes or so, perform another six strengthening exercises or switch to aerobics.

Make sure the aerobic conditioning places you within your target heart rate for at least ten minutes. Subtract your age from 220. Then subtract your resting heart rate. Now multiply by .75. Then add your resting heart rate. The number that results is your target heart rate. Monitor it closely during the course of aerobic exercises, otherwise you're wasting your time.

I would prefer that you strength train to this combination of the two, but many people find it easier to be accountable to a cycle, stair machine, treadmill, or aerobics instructor.

Remember, three workouts per week on alternate days. The duration of the workouts should be from fifteen to not more than forty-five minutes. Beyond that yields no benefit.

Effective exercise and proper eating produce fit and energetic people. It's that simple.

52

Build Muscle to Trim Fat

In the battle of the bulge, or bulges, there is a way to be slimming down while exercising in a manner that most consider bulking up.

You can build muscle to burn fat. This is the central idea of three of my books: *The Nautilus Diet, The Six-Week Fat-to-Muscle Makeover,* and *32 Days to a 32-Inch Waist.*

In ten weeks the average man presented in the Nautilus diet dropped 30 pounds of fat and the average woman almost 19. Those were averages; some lost quite a bit more. In the six-week fat-to-muscle makeover, ninety women lost an average of 12.5 pounds of fat. In the 32-day program, 146 men reduced 17 pounds and trimmed three inches off their waists in a little more than a month.

These people performed circuit strength training for no more than thirty minutes three non-consecutive days each week. They followed moderate-calorie plans ranging from 1700 to 1300 calories per day for men and 1300 to 1000 calories per day for women. Each started at the higher calorie level and descended by 100 every two weeks. The diet was composed of 60 percent carbohydrate, 20 percent fat, and 20 percent protein.

These people built calorie-burning muscle. Each pound they added to their bodies raised basal metabolic rate by an average of seventy-five calories per day. This was in addition to the calories burned during workouts.

Traditional aerobic exercise was not part of the program. These people rested in between workout days so that their bodies could overcompensate for the muscular overload by increasing muscle mass, the process of hypertrophy.

Time efficiency is an attractive aspect of building muscle to burn fat. Ninety minutes of strength training per week will build muscle that burns as many calories during normal activities as hours and hours of aerobic exercise.

But you'd better watch out. Most men trim their waistlines through this strategy while broadening their chest and shoulders.

You can build muscle to burn fat, but you can't be sure that your shirts and jackets will still fit. Not a single person that's been through such a transformation, however, has been displeased with the results.

Decide today that your body needs more muscle, and act on it!

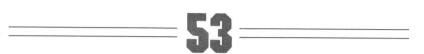

Taking Time to Exercise Keeps Body Ticking

The likeliest excuse we have for ignoring our fitness needs is that we just don't have time.

Most of us are infatuated with our own busy schedules. We're all players in the "I'm busier than you" game, making time constraint a status symbol.

Whatever happened to the leisure class and the idle rich? Lack of available time seems now to be a socio-economic barometer.

Do we control our time, or does time control us?

The other misguided notion about time is that we must not take time for ourselves. Your Good Mother's Badge can be revoked for this, most moms feel.

What would life be like if we didn't take time to bathe?

We find time to shop. Mr. Nielsen tells us we're making time for TV. There seems to be time for the mall or the golf course, and there certainly is no lack of time for eating. Some of us even catch coffee breaks or take a smoke.

A greater percentage of America's corporate chief executive officers (37 percent) exercise regularly than the general population (17 percent). Isn't their time on an hours-per-dollar basis more valuable than ours?

The only thing equal among everyone in this world is the amount of time each of us has every day, every week. We start becoming unequal by how we choose to use our time. Out of 10,080 minutes in a week, couldn't 60 of them be devoted to quality exercise? That is a little more than one-half of 1 percent of our time.

Intense exercise doesn't take up much time. Exercise effect is based on a meshing of intensity, frequency, and duration. This means simply: how hard, how often, how long.

Maximize the intensity, and you can minimize the frequency and duration.

This is a society of microchips and microwaves, in-home shopping, fax machines, drive-through everythings—and yet not time for high-tech exercise!

Time is just like money: you can either spend it or invest it. Spending it moves you toward running out of it. Investing it produces a return.

Time really isn't the question; the question is one of priorities.

A little inner honesty would be enlightening. If exercise is not high enough on our priority list, let's admit it. Let's not hide behind the ludicrous notion that we don't have time for it.

Become a faster reader, and you can do push-ups and sit-ups after reading this article.

Why not invest your time in a quality fitness endeavor? The return will be well worth every minute.

It's Best to Build Strength in Slow Motion

Now that the merits of strength training have been validated by *US News & World Report* and ABC's "20/20," you're ready to pump iron, right?

Minute for minute, progressive resistance training (aka: muscle building) offers a far greater physiological return than all of the aerobic endeavors known to mankind.

But understand what is involved.

♦ Muscle produces force. On its own, muscle does not generate movement, any more than an internal combustion engine propels our cars. Just as our cars move by the engine's force being applied to other com-

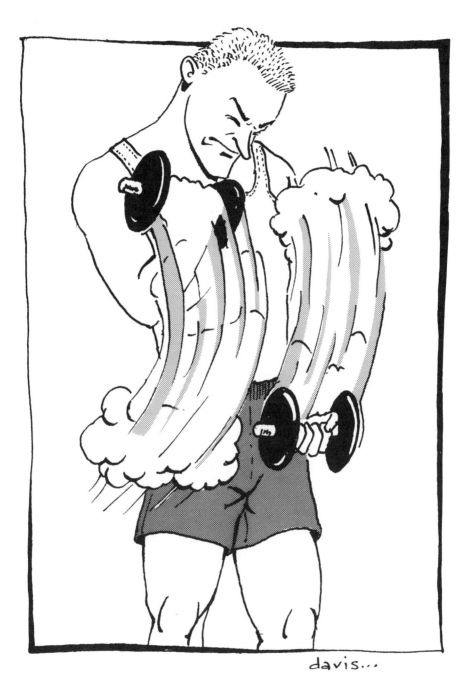

Slow down, you move too fast . . . for better results when pumping iron.

ponents of the chassis, a contracted muscle is linked to skeletal bone by connective tissue. A muscle shortens, it pulls on the bone at a point past a joint. The bones function as levers and the joints as hinges or balls and sockets.

♦ Move slowly to limit momentum and dampen reverberation. To illustrate this point, place the palm of your hand against a wall and push as hard as you can. Now relax and pull your hand back six inches from the wall. Let's suppose (but don't really do this) you were to thrust your hand forward, pushing as hard as you could. The palm of your hand would meet the wall with a thud, resulting in pain and injury.

Using weights or weight machines with fast, jerky, momentum-assisted repetitions damages joints and connective tissue insidiously, if not immediately. If you're currently exercising in this manner, it may be that you're moving your connective tissue closer and closer to the edge. You're going to wake up some morning in pain, not really sure what caused it. Years of jerking weight around will have taken its toll, not via an immediate rip but through accumulated damage.

The safety issue aside, slow, steady repetitions also are more effective because of more thorough muscle fiber recruitment.

Try lifting a weight in a ten-second count. Then lower it smoothly and under control, but less slowly—in about five seconds. Reverse directions smoothly without setting the weight down, and lift again in ten seconds.

Lifting in ten seconds and lowering in five seconds is hard, demanding, grueling, and very effective exercise.

♦ Just as target heart rate is the barometer or training effect from aerobics, degree of inroad into fresh strength is the yardstick of strength training. Unfortunately, this is difficult to measure.

Degree of inroad means that if your fresh muscle can lift 100 pounds, select a weight that's 20 percent less (eighty pounds) and perform slow repetitions until you can no longer lift the eighty pounds.

The difficulty in this is that there's no safe way to measure our fresh strength level. Second, we should perform repetitions until it becomes impossible to move the selected weight. Most of us cease an exercise set when it becomes uncomfortable or difficult—well short of the point of being impossible.

Imagine that there was a gun placed to your head, and you had to do another repetition to keep the trigger from being pulled. That's the type of motivation it takes for effective exercise.

As an alternative to the difficulties of measuring and motivating, we use the progression factor: a little more weight or another repetition at our next workout.

This is okay, but for accuracy the workouts need to be standardized: identical exercises, in the same sequence, with the same time interval between exercise. And then we've got our eating and resting habits, stress level, hormonal factors, workout room stimuli, and a lot of other stuff that mucks up the system.

Did strength training seem simple to you before reading this? I'll spare you a discussion of isolation, range of motion, recovery, ratcheting, and an assortment of other matters you've probably never imagined.

If you've never played golf, the golf swing probably seems simple, too. But a lot of little nuances make a big difference in how the ball travels, and these are not readily apparent to the untrained eye.

The same is true with strength training. If you want to reap its enormous benefits, seek professional help.

55

Three-Minute Workouts Strengthen Your Resolve

As New Year's Day approaches, most of us eat as if we're going to the electric chair on January 2.

If your New Year's Resolution is to get into shape, this is the time to make an Old Year's Resolution: Don't lapse into worse shape.

Prepare for the busy days to come by developing an at-home workout for use in a time-crunch. As little as three minutes of quality exercise is better than none at all. You'd be surprised at what you can achieve in three minutes.

The Slow Squat: Find a place where you're able to stand with something in front of you to hold for better balance. Spread your feet shoulder width apart. You may want to elevate your heels an inch or two by putting a book beneath them.

Keep your back upright (don't lean forward). Slowly lower yourself by bending your knees. Time yourself by keeping an eye on a watch or clock, or at least count at a consistent pace. Try to lower yourself in a legitimate thirty seconds. You should be barely moving.

When you've squatted where your buttocks are a couple of inches from the floor, reverse direction slowly. Do not rest at the bottom. While you're holding onto something—a bedpost, for example—don't pull upward with your arms. Push with your legs, keeping your torso upright.

Make those thighs burn! Take thirty seconds to reach a point where your thighs are at about a 45-degree angle to the floor. Do not straighten your knees; you'll be resting if you do. Once your thighs are at 45 degrees, slowly lower again in thirty seconds.

If you cannot achieve thirty seconds down, thirty seconds up, and thirty seconds back down, just move as slowly as possible and work toward your 30:30:30 goal.

The Slow Push: Lie face down on the floor. Set your hands just outside the shoulders. Push yourself into the UP position—with your arms straight and your body rigid. Start the exercise by bending your elbows to slowly lower yourself to the floor. Keep your body in a straight line from your ankles to your head. Your navel, chest, chin, and nose should touch the floor simultaneously.

Ideally, you've lowered yourself in about fifteen seconds. Don't rest on the floor. Try to push yourself back up as slowly as possible.

If you can't press back up, just reposition yourself to the UP position and slowly lower.

Have you detected a pattern? When you're in a hurry, slow down. Slow repetitions are more efficient.

This time-crunch workout requires only three minutes. That's about the time it takes to draw bath water, warm hair curlers, or heat dinner in the microwave.

For the exercises to be beneficial, however, you must concentrate fully. If this isn't a demanding three minutes, you're either in great shape or you're not following the directions.

56

Negative Training Yields Positive Results

A man in Florida recently retired after winning yet another state weightlifting championship in 1991, and it reminded me of a key component of effective Nautilus training.

Bill Bradford of DeLand High School was named Region III national weightlifting coach of the year. It capped a two-part reign that began in the seventies with six straight state championships.

The significance of his success is the spillover effect it has had on the exercise habits of millions of people. As the DeLand football coach in 1968, Bradford encountered a boastful man who had spent many years in Africa chasing wild animals and building his own exercise devices. The man had an unbending belief in his own method of exercise, which he wanted Bradford to test on his football team.

The man's name was Arthur Jones, and he called his contraption a Nautilus machine. Before the world heard of Nautilus, Coach Bradford was putting it to the test. The Quonset hut at the high school became a Nautilus laboratory. The football field became its vindication.

"Not only were we winning our share," remembers Bradford, "but we were really beating up people physically. We had a game with Cocoa Beach and they lost six or ten players in that ball game. The next week we hurt Melbourne physically. Our kids were strong."

The irrepressible Jones launched Nautilus into national prominence in the seventies, based on two events that originated in DeLand. First, one of the young men training with the new Nautilus devotees, Casey Viator, won the Mr. America title in 1971. Second, when Bradford put together the high school's weightlifting team in 1973, he won 236 matches without a defeat and six straight state championships. Bradford's record was based on technique of performing the lifts, along with strengthening his athletes through Nautilus "negative-only" training. "Negative-only" means the weight is lifted into its top position by a trainer or workout partner. The trainee then lowers the weight under control. When it gets to the bottom, the assistants again lift the weight, and the trainee slowly lowers. "We found through negative-only," says Bradford, "that an individual could handle much more weight than if he or she had done the positive [lifting] movement, therefore activating more muscle fibers."

The coach then adds a disclaimer that is often overlooked.

"There is a fine line," he says, "between how much negative-only training you can take, and how often. Intensity plus rest creates growth. But many people train too much."

Experiment on yourself with chin-ups. See how many times you can pull yourself up from a dead hang. Train for several weeks by performing ten negative-only (the lowering phase) chin-ups. Lower yourself in ten seconds then climb back into the top position by stepping on something or having someone lift you. In a few weeks, see how many times you can pull yourself up. If you're typical, you'll do significantly more.

Bradford, now sixty, was a part of the Nautilus heyday. He worked with everyone from Arnold Schwarzenegger to Eric Heiden, the Olympic gold medal skater, as well as professional football players, bodybuilders, and chief executives from corporate America. About the only sports figures with whom he did not work, incidentally, were the Dallas Cowboys. The organization shied away from Nautilus for many years.

Who knows how many more Super Bowl titles some negative-only training might have produced.

57

Big League Advice: Ease up on Exercise

It is not just coincidence that in the summer of 1990 Nolan Ryan pitched a no-hitter six days after coming off the disabled list. More recently this forty-something-year-old phenomenon won his 300th Major League game.

The lesson to be learned from Ryan's stint of disability is that if he would allow his body more rest, as he was forced to do while disabled with a back injury, he might pitch no-hitters more often and have recently won his 400th game instead of 300th.

Nolan Ryan could be an even greater pitcher.

Examination of his workout regimen shows classic signs of overtraining. That's too much stress placed on his body with inadequate rebuilding periods. Even his pitching coach, Tom House, agrees.

"I'm convinced Nolan has been overtraining all his life," said House.

Ryan's customary routine is an assortment of stationary cycling, sprinting backward and forward, some swimming, heavy-weight work and light-weight work. He also throws a football on the four days in between his pitching assignments.

From a physical conditioning standpoint, Ryan ought to undergo two 30-minute workouts in the standard five-day span between games he pitches. There ought to be at least two good nights of sleep between workouts, and two before he takes the mound for the Texas Rangers.

If he pitches Monday night, for instance, Tuesday afternoon Ryan should do a brisk circuit of approximately ten strength exercises with heavy weights moving slowly through each repetition. One-on-one supervision from a qualified trainer would be a big help.

He should repeat a very similar routine on Thursday afternoon. Basically the leg curl, leg extension, leg press, lateral raise, pullover, and bench press should be performed at both workouts. The arm curl and arm extension should be rotated with the parallel dip, wrist curl, and reverse wrist curl; and the abdominal crunch should be alternated with the rotary torso and back extension.

Plenty of rest on Thursday and Friday and he should be in top form to pitch on Saturday.

A couple of hard, brief workouts in between starts with perhaps some cycling or running on the same days would produce results at least as good in much less time, and probably much better results entirely.

If Ryan is convinced that he must work out every day, then I'd suggest that he do his weight training in a contra-lateral manner. In a contra-lateral program, he would work his right upper body and left lower body on day one after the game; left upper body and right lower body on day two; repeat day one and day three; and repeat day two on day four.

Athletes, coaches, and trainers should understand that too much exercise and too much practice are almost always counterproductive. The human body can be pushed to tolerate many extreme tasks and routines. But it does so at a cost: increased heart rate and blood pressure; joint and muscle aches; stress fractures; headaches; hand tremors; tiredness; irritability; and insomnia.

I don't think Ryan's no-hitter following a stint of disability was a coincidence. The forced rest did him good.

Nolan Ryan should train less, practice less, and rest more.

What's good for Nolan Ryan is good for you—make sure you get plenty of rest between workouts.

58

Haste Makes No Waste In Exercise

A great many people like to rest between strength-training exercises, stocking up on energy for the next round of exertion.

The instantaneous recovery will certainly enable you to lift a greater resistance on the next set, but you've just lessened the efficiency of the exercise.

Unless you're dizzy, lightheaded, or faint, hurry from one exercise to the next, just as if you were a kid at an amusement park eager to get to the next ride.

Total workout time is insignificant; it's the intensity of your effort that matters.

While the exact mechanism for muscular growth is poorly understood, the necessity of intensity cannot be questioned. We must overload the muscle's momentary capability. This means that while we start the set lifting a load that we can smoothly control through a full range of movement, fatigue soon zaps our strength, making movement a demanding challenge.

Resting to gain renewed energy so we can generate movement defeats the purpose of exercise.

When we're trying as hard as we can—and the weight isn't moving—this is overload. Ten to fifteen seconds of trying to lift a resistance that won't budge is the key point of exercise.

At this point we should be breathing like a freight train (never hold your breath). Do not jerk, twist, or relax for a microsecond to get a stretch reflex so we can generate movement through what feels like a little bounce in the muscle.

When you're at the point of overload in an exercise, keep trying as hard as you possibly can, and do not panic if you cannot produce movement. It's desirable that you feel feeble.

If you're breathing and heart rate are so rapid that normal conversation would be impossible (but you shouldn't be talking, you should be concentrating), pace the room for several minutes. When coherency returns, complete your workout, which should consist of twenty to thirty minutes of intensely attacking the major muscle groups.

People can think they're exercising for years and never noticeably improve their physical condition. Unless you achieve overload during an exercise, you've only amused yourself. The only exception is if you're just starting an exercise program.

But anyone who has been training for a couple of months and is halting a set before movement becomes impossible is not realizing the benefit exercise offers.

If the exercise is easy, no amount of it will make a difference. Amuse yourself for hours, and all you'll have to show is a wasting of time.

Twenty minutes of all-out effort will produce far greater results than three or four hours of every imaginable exercise.

Proper exercise, however, does not produce muscular growth on its own. It is only a stimulus. With sufficient recovery time, adequate nutrition, appropriate rest, and maybe even the right hormonal conditions, muscular growth will occur as a response to the stimulus (the exercise).

Again, there is no such thing as a long, hard workout. If the workout was one, it couldn't be the other.

Exercise Takes Mind and Body

While out of town on a business trip, a young man seeks the workout room at his hotel where he is glad to find a stair-climbing machine. For twenty minutes or more, he elevates his heart rate dramatically, his lungs are challenged to their full capacity, and perspiration oozes out of every skin pore.

Once finished, it seems ironic that he would take the elevator back to his room. Yes, after stair climbing to the stars, it was the elevator back to the room.

We have a wonderful way of using modern conveniences to make life easier, and then needing sophisticated technology to make up for the easiness. But this isn't a case merely of a passion for expensive toys. The reality is that the stair-climbing machine captures the imagination, while the stairwell is a bore.

Exercise is a body and mind experience. The body performs at the mind's direction. An unenthusiastic mind will not stimulate the body.

Every exercise method has its legion of devotees.

What captures our imaginations varies with our psychological makeup and personalities. It is important to recognize this, especially if you've been having difficulty with your exercise discipline. The solution is to re-program your mind.

Search out other methods of exercise to see what appeals to you, and search your soul by considering these challenges:

♦ Stop complaining about the rigors of exercise. If you're blessed with a basically healthy body, be thankful that you're able to fatigue muscles and rev up the heart/lung machine.

♦ Focus on the benefits you'll derive from regular exercise, and even visualize attainment of your goal. Keep your eye on the prize not the price.

♦ Read books and articles that inspire and inform. Be consistent and persistent with this reading habit.

♦ Associate with other people who make exercise a priority. They'll influence you toward your fitness goals instead of away from them.

♦ Find a sport or recreation you enjoy and try to improve in it by getting into better physical condition. Remember, however, that you get into shape to play sports; you don't play sports to get into shape.

♦ Recognize that your quality of life depends, in part, on your physical well-being.

♦ In the absence of sophisticated exercise devices, make a game out of the common physical endeavors of life. See if you can reach your target heart rate by raking the lawn. Do floor exercise during your favorite half-hour TV show. Take the fitness trail at a park. Use your imagination.

It's okay to pump iron in the hotel workout room—and then have the bellperson take your luggage to the car. A good workout routine is a controlled, carefully designed strategy period. Carrying luggage is an erratic physical demand that could cause a muscle strain although it shouldn't if you're in good shape.

Weights vs. Wait: Muscle Building for Kids

Should youngsters lift weights? Professional football player Herschel Walker recently said children should avoid lifting weights until they reach age fifteen. "If young people start lifting weights," Walker said, "they can become stiff. They risk losing the flexibility they need for strength and quickness."

I disagree with Walker's rationale and recommendation, here's why:

First, proper weight training—and I emphasize the word "proper"— which I'll get to in a few moments, will increase a youngster's flexibility, rather than impede it.

Second, both strength and quickness are based primarily on the amount of muscle on the body, not the degree of flexibility.

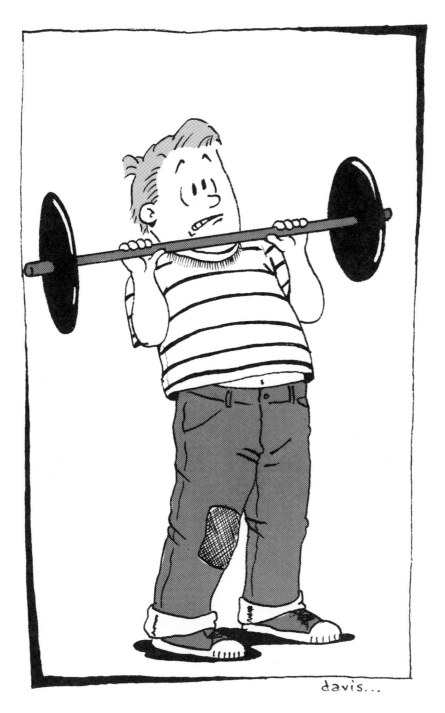

Slow, smooth weight training can be one of the best developmental activities for children.

Third, rather than avoid lifting weights, youngsters should emphasize the activity.

In fact, the American Orthopedic Society for Sports Medicine, after studying the risks and benefits concluded that weight training for children:

♦ Increases muscle strength

♦ Improves motor skills

♦ Protects against injury

♦ Enhances muscle endurance

♦ Has positive psychological benefits

If there are so many benefits of weight training, why has it received a bad review from Walker and some others?

One reason cited for not having children train with weights is that they have not reached skeletal maturity and the growth centers might be damaged. Medical statistics show that 10 percent to 15 percent of all childhood injuries involve the skeleton and 15 percent of those injuries involve the epiphysis (growth plate).

There are differences in immature and mature skeletons. Children's bones are in a dynamic state of growth and remodeling, while adults' bones change much more slowly in response to the stress placed upon them. Keep in mind that the epiphysis is a biomechanically weak area. A sudden force that causes a strain in an adult will often cause epiphyseal fracture in a child.

That's why it is important to understand the difference between weight lifting and weight training.

Weight lifting is a competitive sport in which one attempts to lift the maximum weight on a barbell for one repetition. Olympic weight lifting involves the snatch and clean-and-jerk, and power lifting utilizes the squat, bench press, and deadlift.

Weight training employs barbells, dumbbells, machines, and even body weight in a progressive manner whereby one gradually increases the amount of weight lifted, as well as the number of repetitions.

Weight training should be practiced slowly and smoothly while weight lifting must be performed quickly and suddenly.

Quick, sudden movements are necessary for success in many sports such as football, basketball, gymnastics, and weight lifting. These quick, sudden movements also contribute to and produce injuries.

Youngsters, or even adults, trying to see how much they can lift at one time on a barbell or weight machine are asking for trouble. Instead, they should reduce the resistance and see how much they can lift approximately eight times.

As I've stated in previous books and chapters concerning weight training, for maximum benefits the weight should be raised in a slow ten seconds and lowered in a smooth five seconds. That's ten seconds up and five seconds down. Continue for 4–8 repetitions. When eight or more repetitions are performed properly, increase the resistance by 5 percent at the next workout.

How young is too young? That depends mainly on the child's motivation. I have a five-year-old daughter who often trains with me. About six months ago, she showed interest. So I assembled a small dumbbell that she could hold with both hands for curls, presses, and shrugs. She also does body weight squats, push-ups, sit-ups, and pullups.

I know she is getting benefits from the exercises. But I'm also careful to watch and guide her closely in all her movements. I make sure not to allow her to play with the equipment at any time, especially when I'm not around. And I don't take her to the local fitness center without prior approval.

In the final analysis, weight training is one of the best developmental activities for youngsters—particularly when it is done under trained adult supervision. Stress slow, smooth repetitions—rather than maximum, explosive lifts—and the activity will produce strength, flexibility, and endurance safely throughout the child's body.

61

Preserve Your Muscle Mass

If you're not pumping iron properly, you're getting older faster than you should.

The single most critical step not to just retard, but to reverse, the aging process, according to Dr. William Evans, is strength training.

Dr. Evans, of the U.S. Department of Agriculture's Human Nutrition Research Center on Aging at Tufts University, made this comment during an interview in a recent issue of *Nutrition Action.*

"Much of what we call aging," Dr. Evans notes, "is nothing more than the accumulation of a lifetime of inactivity. Muscles shrink. Body fat increases. The results are an increased risk of diabetes, hypertension, and osteoporosis. By preserving muscle mass we can prevent these problems from occurring."

I agree wholeheartedly with Dr. Evans. But to reap the full benefits from strength training, the lifting and lowering must be performed properly. Plus, the intensity, duration, and frequency of the exercise must be within certain standards.

A recent book of mine, *High-Intensity Strength Training,* describes the salient guidelines as follows:

♦ Lift and lower the resistance smoothly and slowly on each repetition. Do not jerk or throw the weight.

♦ Continue each exercise until momentary muscular fatigue. This fatigue should occur in approximately sixty seconds, or somewhere between four and eight slow, smooth repetitions.

♦ Perform one set of no more than a dozen exercises per workout. In other words, keep your routine hard but brief.

♦ Train no more than three times per week. Your stimulated muscles need time to recover and get stronger.

These are the same guidelines that I applied last fall when I trained Todd Waters for *High-Intensity Strength Training.* Todd, a fitness counselor at the Gainesville Health and Fitness Center, added twenty pounds to his already muscular body in only six weeks. Charlie Baird, a physical therapist at the Florida Sports Medicine Clinic, in Gainesville, Florida, is currently involved in a similar muscle-building program under my supervision. So far, Charlie has packed on twenty-two pounds of muscle in three weeks!

What works for Charlie, Todd, and other strength-minded athletes will work for you—maybe not to the same degree, but still significantly. For it to work efficiently, however, the resistance exercise must be slow, smooth, intense, brief, and infrequent.

When asked specifically about strength training for elderly women, Dr. Evans said, "Women have less muscle mass to begin with, and they start to lose strength more rapidly after sixty. They become so profoundly weak that they have to be institutionalized.

"We hope to keep people independent through strength-training exercise. The National Academy of Sciences said last year that if we can postpone institutionalization of the average elderly person by just one month it would save three billion dollars in Medicare and Medicaid.

"And that doesn't include the savings in dignity and independence for these people."

Start pumping iron seriously—if you're not already doing it. You'll not only put on some valuable muscle mass, but you'll probably live longer.

Keep Your Cool in Light, Loose Workout Clothes

In an effort to "sweat off a few pounds," you put on clothing heavy enough to thwart an Arctic blast. You then stroll merrily along to aerobics class or a circuit of strength training. Lathering up a good sweat will make the flab and the toxins vanish into thin air, you assume.

If you think the barometer of a quality workout is the amount of perspiration you produce, you're in trouble. Your ill-advised strategy is going to produce poor results.

Your body's two million sweat glands are not pipelines to fat stores. Sweat is your body's cooling system. It's like your home air conditioning.

Do you turn your furnace so that your air conditioner has to work harder?

Then why would you wear heavier clothes to hold in additional body heat during exercise?

Wet your finger then blow on it and note the coolness. That's the way sweat cools when it evaporates from the skin.

The sweat produced when you exercise helps maintain optimum temperature for the muscles to function. Heavy clothing hampers the evaporation process. The result is overheating that leads to fatigue, similar to the way your automobile engine shuts down when it overheats.

There are two types of sweat glands, eccrine and apocrine.

The eccrine sweat glands, which are located all over the body, can produce several quarts of sweat per hour during intense exercise or activity. Light, loose workout clothes allow better evaporation. Eccrine sweat, which can also be generated merely by atmospheric temperature in excess of 80 degrees, is nearly pure water.

The other type of sweat gland, apocrine, has nothing to do with temperature regulation. Found in the armpits and about the ears, nipples, navel, and anogenital region, these glands react to stress or stimulation. An odor is produced when apocrine secretion comes into contact with bacteria on the skin.

Sweat is water loss, not fat incineration. The body compensates easily for any fluid loss that is less than two percent of body weight. When water loss from sweat is extreme, however, the fluid surrounding the cells in the body decreases dangerously to low levels. This is dehydration.

You'll have more productive workouts in light clothing. The coolness will enable you to exercise longer and/or harder.

A cool room (76 to 70 degrees) with low humidity and your own light clothing is the ideal exercise environment.

63

Start Now at Becoming Fit for Vacation

Every time I think of family summer vacations, images of Chevy Chase heading for Wally World flood my mind. You remember the movie, don't you? The initial one was titled *National Lampoon's Vacation*, strangely enough, and two sequels, *European Vacation* and *Christmas Vacation,* followed.

Summer vacations are supposed to be the spoils of a year of earnest toil. The accumulated stress of nine-to-five workdays are supposed to dissipate in warm sunsets, cool breezes, and the relaxation of having no demands on our time.

Vacations can be—and should be—a stress relief valve. Since many of us fighting a tendency toward fatness overeat in response to stress, relief should assist our calorie control.

But researchers have found the opposite occurring too many times. People try to cram too much into a vacation. And because they want to maximize their enjoyment, instead of disciplining their eating habits, they seek new kinds of tastebud thrills.

Are you going to bring back excess baggage from your summer vacation? The answer starts with the vacation plan you are probably already making. Here are a few hints.

♦ It is helpful to realize that you'll need a couple of days just to slow down from fast pace. Don't visit every fun park and museum you can.

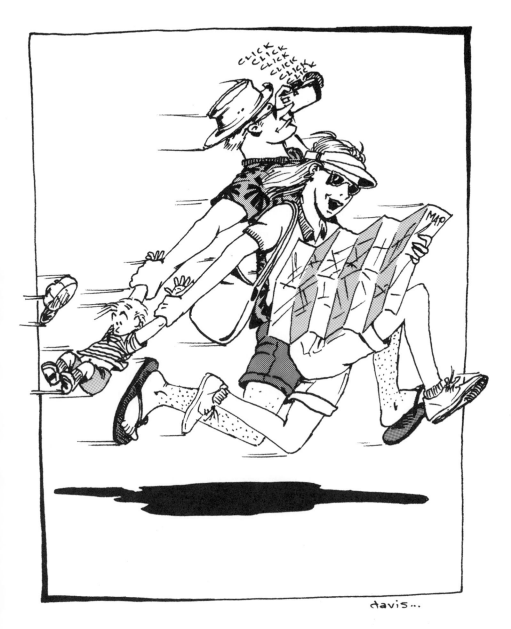

Get into shape for your vacation; do not use your vacation to get into shape!

- Have an activity-oriented vacation. Biking, hiking, tennis, mountain climbing, and so forth are calorie-burning activities that relax and refresh the mind.

- Beware of water sports. Swimming, for instance, is great exercise, but the thermal effect of immersion in water will spur your appetite.

- Cool yourself by drinking plenty of water, instead of sugary sodas or eating ice cream. For a taste sensation use fruit-based blended drinks or juices.

- Don't mistake the dehydration of sunbathing for exercise. Just because you perspire doesn't mean you're burning significant calories.

- Enjoy fine restaurants, but load up on nutrient-dense foods such as salads, vegetables, and broiled fish.

- Set exercise goals for your vacation. Many commercial fitness centers will sell you a pass for a day or week.

- Get into shape for your vacation. Lots of energy will keep you running strong.

- Enjoy alcohol sparingly, if at all.

- Read at least one inspiring fitness-related book.

Do not take these suggestions to extremes. Vacations are memory makers. Their enjoyment is to be relished for years to come. Do not tarnish them by trying to severely diet or become a fitness champion all in one or two weeks.

The battle is one for attaining balance.

Have fun at Wally World!

64

Drink Water When Exercising

When lathered in sweat while laboring under a relentless sun, what should you choose for an energy-boosting, thirst-quenching beverage?

One of the so-called energy drinks? Or simple and traditional H_2O?

Most exercise physiologists have long recommended water as the ideal replacement fluid because it is absorbed more efficiently than any other beverage. That was before the likes of Gatorade, Quickkick, Exceed, and a few others. These specially formulated sports drinks replace the sodium and potassium lost in sweating as well as supply sugar for energy.

There is research that suggests, however, that they provide too much sugar. In a number of studies, researchers have found that beverages containing more than 2.5 percent sugar may hamper performance, particularly in hot weather. Most sports drinks have a sugar content of between 6 and 8 percent. Fruit juices and soft drinks contain even more sugar.

But wait! The latest research—a study using a new monitoring technique—has discovered that although a drink containing 6 percent sugar may leave the stomach more slowly than water, it gets into the bloodstream just as quickly through the small intestine. Endurance athletes experienced significantly less fatigue when they consumed these formulated drinks than when they drank plain water.

Running and other activities that jostle the abdomen also may help process fluids through the stomach more quickly. This permits a concentration of sugar of up to about 8 percent without allowing absorption. (No difference in rate of absorption from one sports drink to another has ever been found in research, incidentally.)

These findings, however, were based on studies using trained endurance athletes exercising for two hours or more. Physiologists do not believe that shorter bouts of exercise require any of the specially formulated drinks.

Water will do—most of the time for most of us. Especially in hot weather, replacing fluid is far more critical than restoring sugar. Eating a few crackers or other high-carbohydrate food should suffice for sugar and sodium restoration.

Whatever your beverage choice, the most important thing, say the experts, is to drink—period. Intense activity in hot weather can produce a loss of more than a quart of water an hour. Neglecting to compensate will result in, at least, lethargy and nausea or even heat exhaustion or heat stroke.

Don't wait until you're thirsty; thirst is satisfied long before you have replenished lost fluids. Cold drinks (40-50 degrees) are absorbed more quickly than lukewarm ones.

In hot weather, consume 16 to 20 ounces of fluid two hours before exercise or activity, and another 8 ounces a half-hour before. While you exercise, drink 3 to 7 ounces every ten to twenty minutes. After exercising, drink enough to replace the fluid you've sweated off (weigh yourself before and after your workout then drink one pint for each pound lost).

Staying hydrated during summer activities will enable you to enjoy them without debilitating repercussions.

SECTION THREE

PERSEVERING

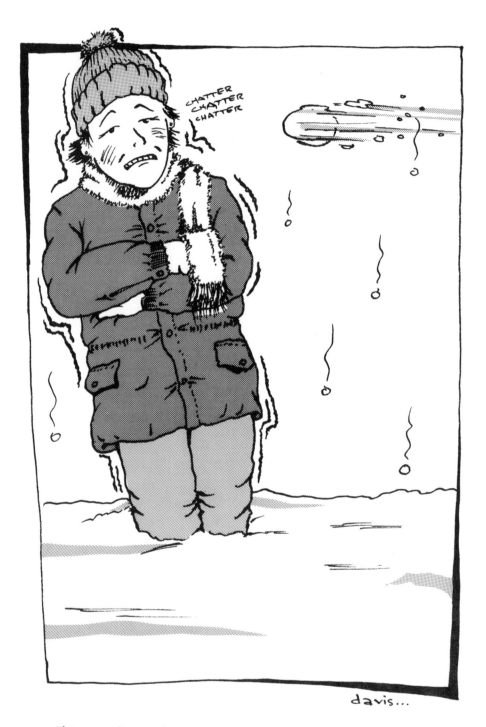

Shivering burns three times as many calories as sweating.

65

Cold Is Hot Way to Burn Calories

There is a simple way to burn extra calories that you've probably overlooked. It's called shivering, which is a lot easier when there's an early
morning chill in the air.

Think of your body as a house. When its temperature dips below the
thermostat, the furnace compensates. Your electric meter records the
energy expenditure which you pay monetarily in the case of your house, or
in calorie burn for your body.

Body temperature is a factor in metabolic rate. Drinking a gallon of
cold water (forty degrees Fahrenheit) requires approximately 226 calories
of heat energy to warm it to core body temperature. Eating a gallon of ice
cream also puts your furnace into overdrive, but ice cream brings with it
more than enough of its own calories for fuel.

To implement effectively the chill factor in your fat-burning efforts, be
sure to use activity and not food to warm your body once it gets too cold.
Warmth is one of the effects of eating. Sometimes we get cold and throw in
a candy bar as another log on the fire. The chill factor will backfire if we're
not careful.

Non-caloric warming measures include sit-ups, push-ups, carrying
boxes, moving furniture, lifting books overhead, performing slow squats,
climbing stairs, walking or a strength-training workout.

If none of these things are possible, hot tea, coffee, broth, bouillon, or
a nutritious soup might help.

There is a theory that repeated cycles of hot/cold produce a thermogenesis effect that accelerates metabolic rate. The utility company will tell
you that keeping your house near the desired temperature generally uses
less energy than letting temperatures drop while you're away and having to
heat it up again.

We can conserve energy—and calorie burn—if we maintain a comfortable body temperature. Think of a calorie as a lump of coal and try not to
conserve but to incinerate as many of them as possible by switching from
heat to air conditioning.

One of the best ways to do this is to take a leisurely walk to warm the
body, then sip a quart of ice water. The walk-then-water strategy is most

advantageous right after dinner. Stop eating when you are no longer hungry—not when you're full.

There are mega-calories between "no longer hungry" and "full." Push yourself away from the table and out of the house for a thirty-minute walk. By the end of the walk you'll realize there had been no need to eat anymore. You would have consumed calories only because you enjoyed the taste of the food and not because your body needed it.

Now that you're back in the house with a warm body, chill it by sipping ice water for the next hour. Ease off the water intake an hour or two before bed, however, or your sleep will be disturbed numerous times.

Sleep slightly cool and you'll have your body's furnace burning up calories throughout the night. Do not use electric blankets or flannel sheets.

The idea of thermogenesis effect may sound a trifle hokey. There is empirical evidence to suggest it works, but guys in lab coats with a lot of initials after their names have yet to test it fully.

If you're only getting fatter while awaiting scientific support, put the chill factor to the test and see what happens.

66

Helping Teens Develop A Good Self-Image

Is there a teenager in your household for whom body image is a painful issue?

The *Tufts University Diet & Nutrition Letter* published a special report recently, and it sounded ominous.

"One of the hallmarks of adolescents, preoccupation with appearance and body image, can wreak havoc on self-esteem. As children reach the teen years, their increased awareness of society's emphasis on having the perfect body, coupled with what is often an acute or exaggerated sense of how their bodies differ from the ideal makes many of them feel worthless and depressed."

Kids today with poor images of their bodies turn to diet pills, diuretics, laxatives, and maybe even anabolic steroids or illegal narcotics. Summer provides more time with your kids, so take advantage of it to find out how your offspring feel about their bodies.

Don't make the mistake of thinking things are the same as when we grew up. A sign of the times is the number of cable TV shows we could find this week that deal with anorexia and bulimia. I don't want this to sound flippant, because cheerleaders and prom queens have killed themselves over an obsession for perfection.

It's a serious situation, and in the next chapter I'll report the warning signs so that you might judge the necessity for seeking professional help.

It isn't just girls, either. Forty percent of twelve- to twenty-two-year-old males at an adolescent clinic in Tacoma, Washington, are unhappy with their weight. One-third say they don't like their body shape. While thin is in for most girls, boys want a muscular, athletic appearance.

The challenge for parents is to find that very fine line that separates sensible attitude from one that is dangerous, and stay on the healthful side of it. Encourage a fitness lifestyle and healthy habits, but discourage fanaticism and obsession.

What do you do with an adolescent who exercises six hours a day and eats little more than celery and carrots? At the other end of the skinfold calipers, what about the child who loads up on milk shakes and French fries and is considerably overweight?

The nourishment we give growing bodies builds the foundation for life. Many experts call osteoporosis a pediatric disease because of a correlation to the lack of calcium (primarily milk) in the growth years.

Iron is also critical during adolescence to meet the needs of growing lean body mass and blood volume and to satisfy the demands of the menstrual cycle. The young lady who shuns iron-rich foods such as lean meat and poultry risks a long-range deficiency.

Of course, teenage girls define "long-term" as the boy who calls next week to ask for a date. Their physical vibrancy upon reaching forty is something they can wait a couple of decades to worry about.

The child depriving himself or herself of food, and the child glutting himself or herself with it, each need to learn about their bodies and nutrition. Of course, nagging probably will backfire. A strong example would be much more effective.

There are many adults who need to learn about nutrition and their bodies. If for no other reason, they need to impart this message to their offspring.

It's a cruel world for fat people, and a dangerous one for both the overweight and the excessively thin.

67

Some Teens Sacrifice Health For a Perfect Body

Body image, self-esteem, nutrition, and the foundation of healthful habits are at stake in every household with a youngster.

Kids with excess fat are easy to identify, and in many respects much easier to deal with. The best parents, however, can overlook the silent agony that lurks inside kids who crave the perfect body and, thus, a perception of a blissful life.

Here are some questions parents should consider:

♦ Does your child exercise regularly and sensibly or obsessively? Can he or she miss a workout without anxiety? Does he or she exercise through serious illness and injury?

♦ Does your child eat in hiding? This could be a telltale sign of binging and purging. If induced vomiting is involved, seek professional medical help immediately.

♦ How frequently does your child characterize herself or himself negatively with an "I'm so fat" or "I'm so ugly" attitude? A little bit is normal, but relentless self-deprecation is a warning signal.

♦ Have you noticed your child possessing diet pills, diuretics, laxatives, anabolic steroids, or other supposed muscle-building concoctions?

♦ Does your child talk incessantly about food and exercise, to the point of ignoring discussion of both more meaningful topics (their education or their future) and trivial ones (the latest ball game)?

♦ Does your child avoid family meals without a reasonable excuse?

♦ Is your child thin and ever trying to be thinner?

An estimated 5 percent of high school girls are victims of anorexia nervosa or bulimia. Seven percent of the boys—and 3 percent of the girls—jeopardize their futures by using steroids. In addition to these, many more adolescents—an estimated 20 percent—suffer from eating disorder symptoms.

The pendulum then swings from the kids who are overly concerned with their bodies to those who never met a cookie they didn't devour.

An estimated 15 to 20 percent of adolescents are considered over-weight. Twenty-two hours per week in front of the TV is not a good slim-ness strategy.

The President's Council on Physical Fitness and Sports tells us that half the girls and a third of the boys ages six to seventeen cannot do a single pull-up. Only 50 percent engage in vigorous physical activity regularly.

Youth sports programs that emphasize winning—at all costs—are ben-eficial to the athletically gifted, but not to the mainstream. If your child shies away from competitive athletics, expose her or him to fitness trails, bike riding, and physical activities with the entire family.

The *Tufts University Diet and Nutrition Letter* suggests making regular family meals a habit, including nutritious items in them, and making every-one participate. For dessert, try a leisurely family walk or bike ride—skip the cheesecake.

A family meal, of course, does not take place in front of "Night Court" reruns or the latest gossip from "Entertainment Tonight." Eat in only one place in your house.

Snacks account for at least 30 percent of teenagers' calories and up to 20 percent of their vitamins and minerals. That's why you need to put low-fat yogurt, fresh fruit, and fortified cereal in places where they're used to finding calorie-dense junk.

If there's any hint of an eating disorder, your family physician should be able to refer you to the appropriate professional help.

68

The Skinny on Gaining Pounds

In our thinness-conscious society, it may surprise you to learn that there are some people who actually need to gain weight. Most of these people are teenagers.

Many teenagers are too skinny for several reasons. One, they have poor eating habits. Two, they have inefficient metabolisms. Three, they are too active.

Here are some basic guidelines for those who want to gain meaningful body weight:

◆ **Get plenty of rest:** Ideally, teenagers should sleep ten hours per night. Keep daily activities low-keyed and at a minimum level.

♦ **Eat a balanced diet:** A nutritious eating plan for one day might include four servings from the meat group, four from the milk group, eight from the fruit/vegetable group, and eight from the bread/cereal group.

♦ **Consume a nutritious breakfast:** Too many teenagers skip breakfast. For gaining weight, a hearty breakfast is a must.

♦ **Select more calorie-dense foods:** High-calorie foods include whole milk, cheese, ice cream, peanut butter, beef steak, safflower oil, chocolate candy, dried fruits, and nuts. (Note: Most of these foods are high in fat, which may elevate a person's blood lipids.)

♦ **Use a blender:** Consuming a blender drink of high-calorie foods is an efficient way to gulp down extra calories. Furthermore, suspending small particles of food in a solution and drinking them speeds up the digestive process. Below are two blender drinks.

Frozen Banana Malt
(595 calories)

1 banana, frozen
1 cup whole milk
1 ounce chocolate flavored
  malted milk powder
1/2 cup vanilla ice cream

Slice the frozen banana and add to the blender with milk and malted milk powder. Turn blender on and mix. Add ice cream and continue to mix until blended.

Peach Shake
(608 calories)

1/2 cup peach nectar
3/4 cup whole milk
1 tablespoon safflower oil
3/4 cup peach ice cream

In a blender mix all of the above ingredients until well blended. Pour into a tall glass and drink.

♦ **Emphasize muscle-building exercise:** When the body puts on weight, that weight can be in the form of fat, muscle, or both muscle and fat. A teenager should be mostly interested in gaining muscle. Stimulating muscle growth requires strength training with barbells or machines.

♦ **Be patient:** Gaining weight for most teenagers will be slow and gradual. This is because the extra calories that are being consumed must be taken into the cells and used to emphasize new tissues. This process takes time. A realistic goal is one-half pound of weight per week.

Smokers—Look at the Facts

Are we immune to the doomsday warnings about cigarette smoking? Every day 1000 Americans give up smoking by being buried.

Every year more Americans die from smoking and tobacco use than all Americans killed during World War II.

Women smokers are more than twice as likely as other women to suffer a disabling or fatal stroke.

Children exposed to their parents smoke have lower levels of HDL (good cholesterol) in their blood; their red blood cells are less able to carry oxygen to the tissues; and their blood contains two toxic chemicals.

Heavy smokers subject themselves to eight times the carbon monoxide exposure allowed in the industry.

Most lung cancer victims die within a year.

Especially alarming are the statistics about teenagers.

♦ American teens spend over $1 billion a year on tobacco.

♦ 60 percent of American smokers start smoking by the time they are fourteen years old.

♦ 80 percent of smokers started smoking by the time they were twenty-one.

♦ About 20 percent of all American high school students smoke.

You've likely heard all this before. We smoke at the expense of our health and our finances.

Thirteen billion dollars is spent each year on smoking-related disease in the United States. If a smoker put $1.50 a day into a savings account at 5 percent interest compounded quarterly the savings would amount to $3079 in five years, $7028 in ten years, and $18,580 in twenty years—not to mention reduced health-care costs.

The Great American Smokeout is fast approaching.

No matter how many times you've tried to quit but failed, try again. "I can't" means only that you're unwilling to do the things necessary to bring about change. You haven't been failing, you've been building a foundation.

Assuming that you are now a pack-a-day smoker, here's the path before you.

If it's been twenty minutes since your last cigarette, your blood pressure and pulse rate have dropped to normal. The body temperature of your hands and feet return to normal.

If it's been eight hours since your last smoke, the carbon monoxide level in your blood has dropped. Your oxygen level goes back up to normal.

Your chance of heart attack decreases if it's been twenty-four hours since your last cigarette.

If you've enjoyed a smokeless forty-eight hours, your nerve endings begin to regrow so sense of smell and taste are enhanced.

After seventy-two cigarette-free hours, bronchial tubes relax and lung capacity increases.

Two to three months of not smoking results in improved circulation, easier walking, and lung function increases up to 30 percent.

One to nine months of not smoking shows marked decreases in coughing, sinus congestion, fatigue, and shortness of breath. Your overall energy level should increase.

Five smokeless years puts a former pack-a-day smoker into a lower lung cancer death rate.

After ten years: precancerous cells are replaced and the lung cancer death rate for the pack-a-day smoker approaches the rate of non-smokers.

Some people, even those well-informed on this issue, decide that a cigarette is worth a six-minute reduction in life expectancy. Too bad they can't derive the benefits they find in smoking in a habit void of devastation.

If you're a would-be quitter, the next chapter might help.

70

Don't Let Your No-Smoking Vow Go up in Smoke

This seems odd, but some people find cigarette smoking relaxing and some are stimulated by it. Others are drawn to the habit of having something to handle, getting a fidget fix I suppose.

Teenagers, perhaps, feel a cigarette presents an adult image.

Some people started smoking for a certain reason but hesitate to quit because they're afraid of gaining weight.

To many, nicotine is strongly addictive.

If you know the hazards of cigarette smoking but have no interest in quitting, don't irritate yourself by reading beyond this point.

You can quit. You just have to be willing to do what's necessary.

There is no disgrace in failing, but failing to try is inexcusable.

Health concerns motivate most quitters. Parents will shed the smoking habit because of the terrible example it sets for their children. Still others get fed up with having yellowed teeth, repulsive breath, cigarette odor in draperies and carpet, holes in furniture, and filthy ashtrays.

Some people hate to think they're dependent on anything, and thus quit smoking to exhibit self-control. Then too, cigarette smoking is associated with a lower rung on the socio-economic ladder. Establish your cause for quitting with written, detailed reasons. Then set a date. Throw a quitting party. Have your drapes and carpets cleaned that day. Make plans for the several weeks thereafter to avoid tempting social environments.

If nicotine gum would help, chew it. Nicotine withdrawal is a struggle. After the first ten days, however, it gets relatively easy. Cold turkey works best. (Reduced tar and nicotine cigarettes are like putting a .22 caliber pistol to your head instead of a .357 magnum.)

If you found cigarettes good for reducing tension, use exercise instead. Physical exertion is a great substitute for a smoke.

A regular fitness program should be scheduled into your normal routine. But also develop spontaneous tension reducers. Squeeze tennis balls in each hand, do some slow squats or push-ups, or perform some isometric exercises.

Even the slightest exertion will hurdle the temptation. There are plenty of things you can do, even while seated at a desk or talking on the phone.

If you need something in your hands, use a pencil, take up needlework, polish your shoes, clean your glasses, or play with rubber bands.

Tape your written list of reasons for quitting to your bathroom mirror. Review it aloud every morning and every night.

You'll also need a written list of things to do instead of smoking.

Don't expect this to be easy. Be sure to discard all your smoking paraphernalia—ashtrays, lighters, everything. Don't store it; pitch it.

Avoid beverages to which you've linked cigarette smoking, at least for a while.

Have plenty of low-calorie food readily available: carrot sticks, celery, apples, fresh ginger, and cloves. These will provide a measure of your fidget fix, and a nice taste in your mouth.

The American Lung Association estimates that only one-third of those who quit smoking gain weight. Another third lose weight, and another third stay the same.

Even if you gain weight, you'd have to gain eighty to a hundred pounds before you'd damage your health to the degree cigarettes do.

Many before you have overcome this disgusting habit, and you can, too. Your heart and lungs will be forever grateful.

71

How to Fix Chuckholes in Road to Perfection

If you need to kickstart your new resolve to improve your eating habits, take the following points to heart:

♦ **Don't try to be perfect.**
Aiming for an impossible task is a sure way to achieve disappointment and frustration. Accept where you are. Be honest about your good points. Give yourself credit. In looking at the entire package of who you are, be proud and thankful of your many fine attributes.

♦ **Identify areas you want to improve.**
The key words in this process are want and improve. Consistent, steady improvement is the goal, three steps forward for every two steps backward—and you will backslide, you can be sure.

If you feel that you have to improve, you probably won't. We tend to rebel against things we "have to" do but if you "want" to improve, you can.

♦ **Be precise and specific.**
Vague generalities of the areas you wish to improve will not zero in on the heart of the matter. For instance, you can't just say that you'd like to improve your eating habits. You must instead write down something precise.

♦ **Prioritize those things you've identified as wanting to improve.**
Trying to tackle them all at once will make the task seem insurmountable. Make a list so that you focus on each item one by one. Get each one off to a good start before starting on the next.

♦ **Be patient, yet persistent; turn frustration into fascination.**
Expect the setbacks that you will unavoidably encounter. You will lapse. You will backslide. You will wander from the course you've mapped out for yourself. When this happens you have two choices to make: **a)** You can use the setbacks as excuses to chuck it all, to give up in frustration, or, **b)** You can turn frustration into fascination. Human behavior is the most complex and compelling issue on planet Earth.

We all do things that do not make any sense, things that are far from being in our best interest. Why? It's all wrapped up in that intricately woven fabric our psyches. Trying to untangle why we do what we do is truly fascinating. We have to learn from our mistakes. Make a plan so that when similar circumstances again arise, you'll deal with them more advantageously.

♦ **Build more accurate associations.**
A fascinating topic that you should learn more about is termed neuro-linguistic programming, NLP for short. This concept has been popularized by Anthony Robbins, a motivational speaker and author.

NLP says that we program our minds through the way that we talk to ourselves. In an oversimplified nutshell, we are overeating because we link comfort, love, reward, security, as a good time to indulge in food and beverage our bodies don't really need.

Tear down harmful associations and build new ones. Link confidence and good health to a lean, well-conditioned body, and place it at the top of your priority list. Deal with your "eating cues" in ways that help attain and maintain your health and vibrancy.

♦ **Continue learning and growing.**
There is no quick fix, no magic potion. The steps above are an ongoing, lifelong process. These steps need to be worked on, nurtured, expanded, mastered, and revised—continually.

72

Tips for Moms Laboring to Get in Shape

The first few weeks after having a baby, particularly your first child, might be the gloomiest a woman will ever experience.

New priorities have slapped you in the face. Your figure is buried beneath a layer of fat, and perhaps your pelvic girdle has been permanently widened. Most pregnancies result in six additional pounds that moms never get rid of.

The baby blues present a formidable fitness challenge.

The psychological boost that can be derived from exercise might be as good an antidote to postpartum depression as the physical refurbishing.

New mothers frequently suffer from pregnancy-related muscle overuse or disuse, general physical weakness, orthopedic injuries, excessive body weight, and Caesarean section recovery problems. They also have a baby (or babies) to tend to, resulting in a lack of sleep and little time for other obligations.

Pregnancy is the greatest athletic event of the typical woman's life. More will be demanded of her body during and immediately after the pregnancy than at any other time of her life, in most cases.

The variables in each situation make it impossible to advise a specific exercise regimen. Your fitness level before pregnancy and what you were able to maintain during it also affect the postpartum plan.

Proceed with caution and with the advice and monitoring of your physician.

You'll have to navigate the turbulent waters you encounter, but we can point your ship in the right direction.

Realize, first of all, that physical strength is extremely important. Carrying a baby, first in the womb and later in your arms, puts a strain on your lower back, abdomen, and upper back.

Your posture and your figure could deteriorate rapidly. Muscular strength must be developed to hold everything in place under the additional load of your new offspring.

Use slow squats to strengthen your legs, trunk curls for the abdomen, pulling motions for the upper back, and very slow, controlled dead lifts for the lower back, along with back extensions while lying prone on the floor.

If you can get to a commercial exercise facility, it should have machines to make your efforts more efficient in each of these exercises. But you can do them at home with little or no equipment. Your weights could be something as routine as water jugs in each hand, and how heavy it feels depends on the extent to which you limit momentum by moving slowly.

Time-efficient exercise features the following:

◆ Slow movement through a full-range motion. How slowly? As slow as you can go without stopping.

♦ Constant tension in the targeted muscle(s). This means no resting points, no relief.

♦ Breathing similar to Lamaze.

♦ Muscle burn. Push through the burn until you absolutely can't stand it. Pretend someone else is paying you $100 per repetition; could you do one more?

The demands of motherhood mean you'll have little time for workouts, so you'll have to maximize the intensity of your efforts. To be effective, exercise must be demanding. Unfortunately, it must result in muscle-burn pain and approach the brink of nausea.

A twenty-minute routine every other day should work fine, as long as you're continually striving for one more repetition, or using a heavier resistance. Your workouts must be progressive.

If you had a C-section delivery, your abdominal muscles need rehabilitation. Ease into trunk curls slowly and cautiously, once your doctor has given permission to begin. Perform each one with a methodical slowness.

Don't expect to feel like exercising, but do it anyway. A lot of times after pushing yourself to get started, you'll notice the exercise makes you feel better.

You'll be more successful if you set a regular time to exercise and make every effort to stick to it.

On eating, you may have developed some bad habits under the immunity of maternity clothing. Salads, soups, and fruits should make up eighty percent of your daily calories until the unwanted pounds depart at a rate of two pounds per week.

With persistence, patience, and a positive outlook, you should be able to recapture the figure and vitality you once had.

73

Deprive Yourself of Body Fat

As I write this there is a chocolate brownie with peanut butter dripped on top calling my name from beneath the plastic wrap my friend draped over a plate of these delights in the kitchen.

We're awaiting company. Should I violate my friend's "no touch" proviso, I'll be writing the rest of this chapter with fewer fingers with which to strike the keyboard of my computer.

I'm really feeling deprived. That brownie wants me just as much as I want it. It's looking for a home on my waistline.

Diet practitioners contend the failing of most diets is that they leave people feeling deprived. By that reasoning, I should go claim my prize. But wait! The diet guru will tell us to eat something healthy for the body. Then you won't feel deprived.

Somehow, a carrot stick won't do when the juices of my mouth are crying out for the sweet melody of chocolate and peanut butter.

What a dilemma. As much as I would enjoy the taste of the brownie, however, I'm not eager to add it to the collection of fat cells that bulge out over the top of the belt.

I'll just have to endure feeling deprived, and so will most of you if you desire a body that is not fatter than makes you happy.

Beware of the diet counselor who says you won't feel deprived if you follow the regimen they recommend. Learn to deal with seeming deprivation, instead of the hocus-pocus of dancing around it.

If you're going to lose weight, you're going to feel deprived at times. If you're going to get into shape, you're going to feel muscle burn pain and fatigue at times. There is no easy, painless way of achieving these goals.

Whatever your aim, you have to deny yourself many things in order to achieve it. This self-denial, however, is really an exchange of something to get something else. We make our choices based on a hierarchy of values.

Andrew Carnegie taught us the law of increasing returns. To understand this, think about a farmer who plants a bushel of seed. After the soil, the sunshine, and the rain have worked their magic, what the farmer harvests is not just a bushel of seed. If that's all he were to get back, the farmer would never have planted the seed. He gets back hundreds of thousands of bushels of grain.

Deprivation, denial, and self-discipline are concepts we're not eager to embrace. But they become more palatable when we think of them in a term that we like—investment.

Deprivation is only a temporary thing. Implemented correctly, we will someday harvest our ultimate goal.

Temporarily denying ourselves whatever is in the way of our goals produces an end result that makes the discipline worthwhile.

Deprivation in a weight-reducing effort is only temporary. It's only temporary because as you master saying no to cravings, the task becomes less difficult. With each success, you harness power and build confidence. Correspondingly, your body gets into a position where it can stand a brownie now and then without inciting an ugly collection of fat cells.

So I'm willing to deprive myself—temporarily. The company will be here pretty soon, after all.

===================== **74** =====================

Undissolved Vitamins Still Unresolved Problem

One man says an X-ray of his stomach showed a multivitamin pill in pristine condition. Another man claims he found a layer of vitamin pills in the bottom of his septic tank.

The chairman of the Department of Pharmaceuticals at the University of Maryland has been looking into the problem of undissolved vitamins for several years.

This man, Ralph Shangraw, says that in 1986 "more than half the calcium supplements in the marketplace failed to disintegrate within thirty minutes."

The problem is that "if a calcium carbonate tablet doesn't disintegrate by the time it leaves your stomach, chances are it won't get absorbed in your bloodstream," says Shangraw.

Even if vitamins and minerals disintegrate, they still might not get into the bloodstream. If they don't disintegrate, you can be sure they won't.

Drugs must either disintegrate or be at least 50 percent or 75 percent dissolved after being agitated in simulated stomach or intestinal juice for a specified length of time. There are no such tests for vitamins and minerals, however.

Why are some of our vitamins and minerals passing through our system like marbles?

Some companies compress them too hard to make them small and easy to swallow. Some companies remove starch so they can make a "no starch" proclamation on their labels. Many companies give tablets a shellac coating, which resists stomach acid.

When acacia gum became scarce, companies switched to a more acidic gelatin. When mixed with calcium carbonate, this results in something resembling cement.

U.S. Pharmaceutical (USP) standards exist, but compliance is strictly voluntary.

There is no need for a vitamin or mineral dosage that exceeds 100 percent of the Recommended Dietary Allowance. Many people use vitamins as magic pills, mistakenly believing that they assure good health. Assuming that the vitamin gets into your bloodstream, the excess simply passes through.

Dissolvability is not a problem with tablets containing only vitamin C or the B vitamins, incidentally. And vitamin E capsules dissolve more easily than vitamin E tablets.

Many people who suffer a lactose intolerance rely on calcium tablets, which has the problems mentioned above, but there are questions, too, about niacin. A test of five brands of sustained-release niacin tablets showed that two were not even half-dissolved in twelve hours.

Questions also have been raised about vitamin potency. Some supplements are difficult to formulate. The components react with each other and decompose over time. The Food and Drug Administration recalled twelve defective supplements in 1989.

So, what are we to do?

♦ If you're taking calcium, check the label or call the company to see if the supplement meets USP's dissolving tests.

♦ If you take niacin, take several smaller doses rather than a sustained-release tablet.

♦ Only buy supplements that have expiration dates.

♦ Increase your chances of ingesting a high-quality supplement by sticking to name brands.

75

Take the Strain off Your Lower Back

If you haven't seen a doctor concerning low back pain, you stand a one in three chance of doing so sometime in your life. Low back pain is as common as the pain-relieving medications many of us buy at the drugstore to combat it.

Most of us do not exercise our spine's full range of motion on a consistent basis, and few of us relax our spine, even when we are not moving. Our modern lifestyle itself is generally a backache waiting to happen. We may be sitting at a desk or in a car, but stress on our nervous system keeps our muscles taut, squeezing off the nerves' pathways.

But this is just one phase of the malady. Come Friday at 5:00 PM, we transform our couch-potato lifestyle into that of weekend warrior. Monday, therefore, is the busiest day in a chiropractor's office, treating those who abruptly shifted from neglect of their spine to the abuse of it.

Back pain often is debilitating. Further, the more we sit, the more we eat. The result is that we amass fat and waste muscle. And even though we'll likely find temporary relief from the discomfort in our backs, a fatter and weaker future is the breeding ground of more back problems.

Low back pain needs to be either cured or prevented, and many of the common causes are within our control. Here's a checklist to see whether you can take some strain off your spinal column.

♦ **Posture.** Any posture which compromises the natural curvature and muscular balance of the spine places strain and tension on the supporting muscles and ligaments, weakening them. Without proper support, the joints of the vertebrae are forced to carry weight they are not meant to carry. This leads to premature spinal degeneration and pain.

♦ **Over-exertion.** We tend to ignore the subtle signals our back gives us. In spite of a little twinge here or a spasm there, we continue to move furniture, perform yard work, or sit at a computer for endless hours. The result is a strained muscle or a squeezed disc.

♦ **Emotional stress and muscular tension.** Stress causes muscles to contract. Chronically contracted muscles stop the circulation of blood and oxygen. The result is pain and atrophy in the muscle and misalignment of the joints.

♦ **Degenerative wear and tear.** Although the spine undergoes a natural aging process, inappropriate alignment and poor use of the spine can accelerate that process. Arthritis, osteophytes (bony growths around the vertebral bodies and facet joints), osteoporosis, disc aging and facet joint damage are some of the effects of aging that can cause low back pain.

♦ **Herniated disc.** A herniated or protruding disc can cause severe back pain, but only a small percentage of back pain can be attributed to this condition. Pain usually accompanies a herniated disc only if the escaped disc material is bothering a nerve.

♦ **Structural abnormalities.** Occasionally, low back pain is caused by a predisposing condition such as scoliosis, spina bifida, or spondyfolisthesis. These abnormalities will be apparent on an X-ray.

♦ **Trauma.** Automobile accidents, work-related mishaps, and sports injuries can damage the soft tissue or the bony structure of the spinal column, or both.

Stretching and strengthening your muscles is the best protection you can give your spine, along with some common sense in what you ask it to do.

Don't just play sports and think the activity will avert low back pain. At some point, it is likely to cause the pain. As stated many years ago by Dr. Fred Allman, a one-time president of the American College of Sports/Medicine, "Don't play sports to get into shape. Get into shape to play sports."

76

Golf Swing Can Sometimes Be a Pain

A golf swing can be a terrible thing to do to your sacroiliac. This joint is the junction of the arrow-shaped bottom part of the spinal column and the hip bones (iliac).

A golfer's forward lean combined with the rotation of the hips and lower back during the typical golf stroke places a great deal of stress on this critical area.

Weekend golfers should take note of the exercise trailer that travels the Professional Golfer's Association tour. Pros like Payne Stewart, Fuzzy Zoeller, Jack Nicklaus, Curtis Strange, and Bernhard Langer have all suffered low back pain in recent years. That's the reason fitness equipment is always nearby.

Many ligaments bind the lower spine (sancrum) to the hip bones (ilium) on each side. The relative immobility of the joint and the abundance of ligaments in the area, combined with torso rotating or twisting, causes frequent ligament strains.

Coming out of nerve roots in the area is the sciatic nerve, the largest and longest nerve in the body. The sciatic nerve sends signals through the

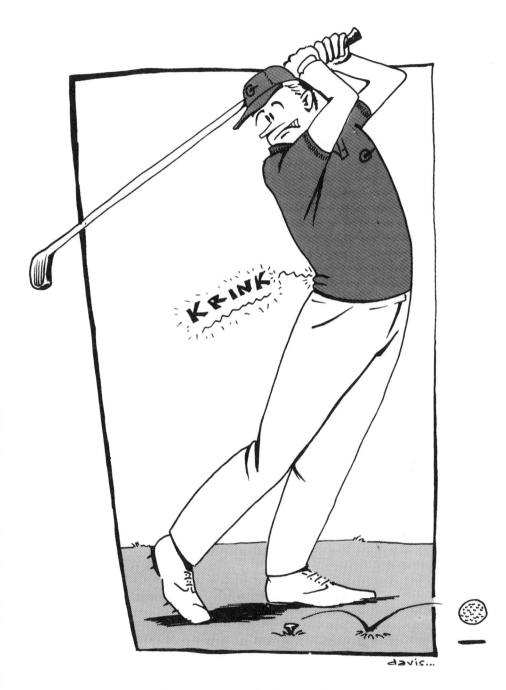

Strength training can help your lower back
as well as your golf game.

buttocks region (gluteal), down the structures of the back thigh, through the entire leg, and into the foot. It receives sensation back along the same route.

Except for the gluteus maximus, the sciatic nerve runs over the surface of the buttocks muscles. It is easily affected by strains to the ligaments of the sacroiliac joint.

Sciatic pain is often an example of referred pain, meaning that it is felt some place other than where it originates. When a disc in the lower part of the back presses on the sciatic nerve, or when a sacral ligament is sprained, you can feel pain as far away as your toes.

Pain in this area is by no means exclusive to golfers. So here are a few safeguards that may save you a lot of misery.

If no exercise equipment is available to you, lie flat on your back with your knees bent and your feet flat on the floor. Push your pelvis upward by pressing with your legs. Your shoulders and upper back should remain flat against the floor. Perform several of these pelvic tilts.

Again from this position, clasp your hands on the back of one thigh and pull toward your chest as tightly as you can while keeping your low back flat on the floor. Alternate legs several times, and then do both at the same time.

Another exercise is just to stand on one foot next to a table, and swing your free leg back and forth slowly from the hip. Be sure to press backward as far as you can so that your buttocks muscles tighten fully.

Proceed very cautiously with any bending exercises, such as deadlifts. Move very slowly and very smoothly. It should take you ten to fifteen seconds to go from as far forward as you can bend to standing straight up.

These exercises can add strength and flexibility, but there's no guarantee that a golf swing or any other activity won't produce an injury.

Sciatic pain signal is usually a pins-and-needles type of feeling and numbness. When sciatic pains caused by strain of the sacroiliac ligaments, or a misalignment of the joint, manipulation of the joint can be of great help. When it is caused by a protruding disc in the lumbar spine, an adjustment can also help.

A chiropractor may be as important to your golf game as a caddle.

Duffers should also note the following:

♦ Cut down on your back swing and follow-through.

♦ Avoid lateral bending by keeping the shoulders over the hips throughout the swing.

♦ Flex the knees and avoid excessive bending while putting.

♦ Instead of bending over, squat, so that your legs take some of the burden off your low back.

The best advice, however, is what you've been striving to do anyway—become a better golfer. When you cut down on your strokes, you lessen all kinds of strain.

77

Learn to Exercise Good Habits

There's a television commercial with a slogan that should be applied to our eating and exercising habits. It's the high-energy Nike commercial punctuated by the phrase, "Just do it."

You've seen these commercials. Many of them feature Bo Jackson, the once dual professional baseball and football player.

The commercials show snippets of physical activity with little or no narration, climaxing in a flash of "Just do it."

The company's goal must be to make us wear out our sneakers quickly so we have to purchase another pair. Whatever their objective, their psychology is refreshing.

You don't like to exercise? Too bad.

Can't follow a sensible eating plan? C'mon!

Just do it.

Our ability to rationalize is highly counterproductive. A long string of excuses can be linked together so that we're satisfied with just about anything.

A recent telephone poll of 1220 adults shows that 11 percent think their physical conditioning level is excellent while 58 percent think it is good.

Responding to this survey, Steven Breckler, an assistant psychology professor at Johns Hopkins University, said that such studies "find that people perceive themselves in favorable terms, and usually in more favorable terms than the facts would warrant."

Do we want to believe we're in better shape than we really are? We must, or we'd be more diligent in adhering to a fitness lifestyle.

Usually procrastination is involved. We're going to improve our habits—someday, but not today. Today the conditions are not right. We'll be better able to tackle the situation at some undefined point in the future.

This is our nature. It's also our handicap. We reside in a high bracket of self-indulgence.

How do we break free? How do we bring to a screeching halt the vicious cycle we are in and shift into a new direction?

There are countless hurdles. Our habits have been constructed over a lifetime. They won't easily loosen their grip.

When we make an attempt and then are faced with a deviation from our normal routine, there's another excuse to cast discipline to the wind.

We can fool ourselves into thinking just about anything. When the task seems insurmountable—just do it.

Isn't all the thought and analysis we want to put in to the deep-seated reasons just a stall tactic?

Does TV shape our attitudes, or is it a reflection of them? Either way, its influence is powerful. Most TV commercials provide inducements to consume high-calorie foods and beverages. These sneaker commercials excluded, TV watching is hazardous to our waistlines. Studies show TV watchers tend to be fatter than those who are "just doing it."

Which are you going to be?

78

Poor Attitude Toward Bad Habits Is Criminal

Do you know that many criminals are convinced they've done nothing wrong?

"I have spent the best years of my life giving people the lighter pleasures, helping them have a good time, and all I get is abuse, the existence of a hunted man."

That statement is the expressed sentiment of Al Capone, as reported in Dale Carnegie's classic *How to Win Friends and Influence People.*

Talk to any prison inmate and you're likely to detect some fallacious reasoning for their anti-social behavior. They consider themselves—at worst—victims of an unfair system.

If heinous criminals aren't convinced their behavior is inexcusable, then how are we to face up to addressing our fitness needs?

A few too many nachos is more socially acceptable than a machete murder, we'll all agree. The point of this comparison is that our human minds are capable of rationalizing so that we can justify any of our actions, or inactions.

Do you know that half of the heart-attack victims who smoked previously resume the habit? In many cases they're not even determined enough to improve their cholesterol level, despite the undeniable correlation. Repeat heart attacks are common, especially if you smoke and/or have high cholesterol. A great many heart-attack victims also neglect regular exercise.

Many times the second heart attack is fatal. In fact, if you're a male who has suffered a heart attack and your cholesterol level is above 240, you stand a 20 percent chance of dying within ten years.

Do you know how often I've heard the "I'm going to die anyway" attitude? Apparently, there's no reason to postpone the inevitable, or to enhance the quality of the time remaining, or to spare loved ones premature grief.

Isn't this just about as absurd as Al Capone thinking he was basically the kind of guy you'd invite to Rotary?

Pointing out where other people think irrationally is far easier than recognizing our own misguided reasoning. Certainly if Al Capone could justify his actions, there are plenty of excuses for poor eating habits and a sedentary lifestyle.

What does it take to convince people to change? If the first heart attack isn't reason enough, what words can be written to avert ending doom?

Don't smoke, eat properly, and exercise effectively. There are no excuses.

In many instances, fitness is an issue we intend to deal with later, sometime in the future, when we feel conditions will be perfect. Funny how that time never arrives.

More people are out of shape than are in shape because it's easier to be out of shape—just do nothing. But it's far more rewarding to be in shape.

If you're not the type of person who values an energized, fit body, change. Be willing to break out of your existing comfort zone.

The first thing you might do is write down why you would like to be in shape. Explain how you would like your life to be different based upon enhancing your health and fitness.

The next step is to visualize attainment of your goal. See yourself in more stylish clothes or excelling at your favorite sport. Start to imagine the confidence and pride you'll have in yourself.

Don't let your attitude about fitness be as deviant as Al Capone's concerning law and order. Stop deflecting all the health and fitness messages. Let at least some register, and take the appropriate action.

Begin today.

79

Buddy System Helps in Fat Fight

Shedding body fat permanently is an almost-brutal discipline. It's not a question just of what we eat, but also what we do, how we feel, where we go, and what activities we engage in. We have to modify our total life—for good—or the pounds will return.

Modifying our lives to this extent requires the help and cooperation of those around us. The biggest part of most of our environments is that person we took vows with some years ago, our spouse. This article concerns a cornerstone of successful lifestyle change—spousal support. It also takes the woman's perspective; meaning that it's about the role of the husband in a woman's effort to regain the figure she had on her wedding day.

Husbands have to help. They have to lend strength to the cause. They have to be cheerleaders. They have to notice and praise. They have to look for ways to help reduce stress. They have to give up most of their own gluttony.

"Being a woman is a terribly difficult task since it consists principally in dealing with men," wrote Joseph Conrad.

Nothing other than gentle, encouraging words should pass from hubby's lips. "You've lost weight," is food to the ears instead of food to the mouth. Praise the effort your wife is making, even if the results come slowly. The critical time is when there is a backslide. No kicking while they're down. The attitude to express should be one of lending a hand for your wife to pick herself back up.

Fattening foods the wife craves can't be kept in the house, even though hubby and children may want them. Everyone has to make changes. The total environment has to be different from what it was, elevating health and fitness several notches on the priority list.

Going out to dinner has to be different. Old favorite restaurants where you would indulge without end have to be avoided for a while. Go to new places where you each have arranged a sensible selection. Alcohol will kill any fat-loss effort, so avoid it while the wife is trying to lose.

Don't insist on doing things that will spur your wife to overeat. Help her establish more healthful habits.

Battling frumphood can be a crisis. Do not underestimate the effort permanent lifestyle changes require. The immediate surrounding environment has to adopt a new attitude, and a wife and mother's world encompasses husband and children. All have to help.

Anyone attempting lifestyle change needs people around them who understand the importance of their goals. Loved ones have to share anxiety and worry so that the dieter doesn't turn to eating to alter her feelings.

Two books by Gary Smalley, *The Joy of Committed Love* and *Love Is a Decision,* might help. Smalley writes about the family and interpersonal relationships and says:

"If a couple has been married for more than five years, any persistent disharmony in their marriage relationship is usually attributable to the husband's lack of understanding and applying genuine love."

Excess body fat can be emotionally based, you know. Our loved ones have to be our allies.

80

The Benefit of Avoiding The Consequences

The best thing you can do to get into superb physical condition is not pumping iron, sweating to Richard Simmons' oldies, swimming, starving, or eating sensibly.

The indisputable action you must first take is to identify the reason you want a body like Madonna's, the energy of a teenager, and vibrant health that will carry you through a rich and rewarding life.

Without a reason, there is no vehicle that will transform you into a fitness champion. Half-hearted attempts at anything produce little.

Jane Fonda has a reason. So does Arnold Schwarzenegger. We might find some reasons, too, if we search deeply.

Let me tell you about a woman whom I'll call Betty.

Betty has been involved in a fitness program for quite some time, deriving only partial benefit. It's kind of like having a computer that's capable of elaborate number crunching, desktop publishing, compounding interest, tracking investments, automating bill payments—and all you can do with it is play computer games.

Betty has been casually going about her fitness program—particularly the eating component of it—for quite some time. Suddenly, she has come face to face with a reason for getting serious.

Her class reunion is six weeks away. Her tone of voice was desperate when she said, "I can't go there looking like a fifty-year-old."

Unfortunately, she won't have class reunions every week, so her reason is likely to fade seven weeks from now unless she learns a lesson.

Everything we do requires a reason. We even have to have a reason for getting up in the morning.

All of our actions are governed by the desire either to gain pleasure or to avoid pain. We are always subconsciously evaluating benefits and consequences. Do you know the distinction?

A benefit, for example, is if I offered you $100,000 to run a mile in five minutes. You'd give it a try, right? You'd start off running as fast as you could, dreaming of what you'd do with $100,000.

At the point, however, where your heart-lung machine began pounding like a bass drum and you felt as if somebody has poured gasoline down your throat and lit it, you'd say the heck with the money. You never had it anyway, so you haven't lost anything.

You missed out on the possible benefit. You were motivated to try, but your threshold was not that great.

Let's change this scenario slightly. Let's suppose your child was one mile away, playing on a train track. You could see your child, and you could see a train coming, about five minutes and five seconds away. Now, could you run a mile in five minutes?

It's safe to say that you could, or you would kill yourself trying. There was a consequence to not running a mile in five minutes.

That's the difference between benefits and consequences. A benefit is gaining pleasure. A consequence is avoiding pain. We do much more to avoid pain than we do to gain pleasure, meaning that our consequences are more profound to us than our benefits. There are countless examples of this in everyday life.

Betty has had plenty of time to realize benefits from her fitness program but only now does she see a consequence.

We all have reasons to keep our bodies functioning at a high level, but we ignore them.

Maybe the best reason is that if we don't do something to keep ourselves in shape, there certainly will be consequences eventually. And a lot of times that consequence can be more dire than a class reunion.

81

Have Good Things in Mind for Your Body

Potato chips and a soft drink for breakfast. A morning snack of ice cream with chocolate syrup. Lunch of a bag of cookies, and dinner consisting of peanuts and beer.

You would recognize the effects on your physical well-being, I presume, if the above represented your daily food intake. The cellular structure of your body would not exude health and vitality, nor would you likely be very lean or muscular.

Have you ever considered the nourishment you give your mind? Are you making your mind healthy and strong, or are you allowing it to be gunked with junk?

Particularly inside the fat-loss arena, most of us wire our minds so that it's difficult to feel good about ourselves, and very easy to feel badly. We impose limitations with negative self-talk, the likes of "I can't do this or that" or "I'm no good at that" or "I'll always be fat."

Such statements are our mind's equivalent to a steady diet of potato chips, candy bars, peanuts and soft drinks.

Negative self-talk is a part of a defense mechanism we develop to protect us from having to experience what we anticipate will be unpleasant feelings or emotions. Before making a decision, we test the waters to see what it would be like if we really did commit ourselves.

This phenomenon, emotion-reaction thinking, leads to negative self-talk. Because a past experience evokes a certain feeling, we're afraid that anything similar will again produce bad feelings. So we feed our mind with excuses that reduce dreams into useless, idle wishes.

Genetic factors aside, a lean, attractive, well-conditioned body begins with a mind programmed to make it happen. The problem with your waistline starts at the control center in your head.

The solution lies in awareness, recognition, and strategy.

Are you aware of this problem? Are you feeding your mind for fat loss?

The excuses have to stop somewhere. You can recognize negative self-talk by its emotional energy.

There will be lag time between the outburst and your recognition of it. Once you've pinned down when it happened, go back and analyze the thoughts and conditions that preceded it.

As we begin to better understand our reasons for negative self-talk, we'll find ourselves recognizing it more readily.

Eventually, we'll learn to recognize and stop these powerful negative suggestions before they unleash their destruction.

We have the ability to choose the feelings and emotions we experience. We do this by placing appealing thoughts and images into our subconscious mind.

Visualization is an effective technique for this. The best time for visualization is when your mind is in that dreamy state between sleep and awake, usually in bed in the morning or evening.

Create an image in your mind of the way you want to look or act. Imagine it in detail, making it as realistic as possible.

You'll get better at visualization with practice. Just like you don't play golf very well the first time you hold a club, don't expect awesome impact from visualization on your first try. Persevere and it will pay off.

Your mind is a powerful tool that should be used constructively. Computer programmers know about "garbage in, garbage out." That microchip that directs your life needs healthy input.

If you feel you're overweight, start feeding your mind for fat loss.

82

Looks Can Be Deceiving Even to Yourself

On a scale of one to ten, rank your body's physical attractiveness. Place a number on how, in your mind, your contour, dimension, and shape measure up to the standard you set for yourself. Before reading any further, give yourself a ranking.

If you're the typical woman, you probably feel that your hips are too wide, thighs too flabby, or your tummy features an ugly bulge. Men usually have what we might affectionately call a big gut, or a roll of fat more to the side of the waistline, alias a spare tire.

Only a small number of us take any consistent action to do anything about it, but our bodies bother most of us. We are actually afraid to accept or like our bodies, at least the way they are right now.

We dream of that point in the future where we will really get serious, be motivated and light a fire for fitness.

You probably think that next you're going to read a call to action and an admonishment against making excuses. But more than fire and brimstone, let's talk about compassion.

Some people, especially women, spend much of their day dealing with food: shopping, budgeting, planning meals, cooking meals, and cleaning up the kitchen.

For people who perform these duties, food never really leaves their minds. They simply go from eating food to thinking about food until they're eating food again.

The power of suggestion was clearly demonstrated to me at a seminar on cardiopulmonary risk factors. The seminar wasn't ten minutes old when a man went into cardiac arrest.

If you deal with food all day, a good deal of it is going to work its way into your mouth.

If you can't stay on a so-called diet, don't assume that you lack strength of mind.

Most of the time we apply restrictions for achieving body fat reduction—a long list of food that we cannot eat. Whatever we're told not to do our minds tend to dwell on doing. More than being a question of having willpower, fitness frustration can be a glitch in your strategy.

Consumption of calories is a large issue in most of our lives. Food has turned into a companion for many of us. The chemical changes that occur with the ingestion of food diminishes anxiety. That is why so many of us eat when we get frustrated or stressed.

Repressed emotions find an outlet, and often that outlet is food.

Don't look for an external solution to your internal relationship with food. Find out what's eating you, and then maybe you'll be able to enjoy food without being controlled by it.

An eating diary or journal is the best instrument for getting a handle on this situation. Such record keeping reveals our inner chatter. Once aware of what's going on, we are then able to deal with it.

Make sure your journal keeps track of and records the events and feelings—past and present—that fuel your eating practices. But it should also offer you a place to cheer yourself on. It is a laborious task, but the diligence you exercise in keeping an eating journal or diary will be generously rewarded.

The only criterion governing our eating should be the care of our body. The care primarily should be based on health concerns, not achieving a certain physical image.

Do you feel like you're really not heavy, but you've never been thin enough?

Such an impulse is the warning signal that you should be grateful for what you've got, instead of crabbing that you haven't lately been mistaken for a fashion model or an Olympic athlete.

We are afraid to like our bodies. How did you rank yours? If you're typical, you ranked it too low.

We're afraid that if we like our bodies, we'll lose the drive for self-improvement. If we dislike our bodies, we're inclined to push ourselves to punishment, although a demanding workout isn't punishment, it's an investment.

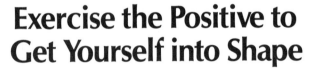

Exercise the Positive to Get Yourself into Shape

Do you find yourself asking, "Why am I so fat?" or "Why can't I ever get into shape?" These kinds of questions—inquiries that your brain takes seriously—assure that you will always be fat, and never be in shape.

How we talk to ourselves makes a difference. This is because the brain is like a computer. When you give it a command, it searches its data base for a response.

If you want confirmation of why you're fat and out of shape, your data base probably has plenty of reasons and excuses in storage.

You're fat because you love the taste of rich, creamy sauces and cheese, for instance. You link the taste of the cheese with something wonderful. The result is that you head for the instant happiness and satisfaction of the taste of the cheese. Your brain has responded to the question it was asked.

You can't ever get into shape, because your brain reminds you that it's easier to lounge on the couch or stay in a warm bed a half-hour longer in the morning.

If you want to be in shape, a healthy first step is to change the questions you set loose in your brain. Remember, the brain's intuitive powers aren't what you might think. It doesn't understand that "Why am I so fat?" really means "I'm sick and tired of being fat. What can I do to change it?" Precision is a must in the wording of your questions.

Think about the fact that the quality of our lives is equal to the effectiveness of our communication, with ourselves first and foremost. If you're having trouble grasping this, think about the following:

What is the typical explanation for an argument or disagreement with another person? Hasn't a "lack of communication" achieved the status of a wornout refrain? More precisely, this lack of communication is actually poor communication.

The messages running through our own minds, although never verbalized to another human being, trigger actions at the subconscious level. Our internal communication is vitally important.

Tony Robbins explains this in much greater detail. Robbins writes books such as *Unlimited Power* (Fawcett Columbine, 1986) and cassette tape programs such as "Personal Power" (Robbins Research International, 1989).

So, instead of "Why am I so fat?" it's better to ask, "What actions can I take today to get myself into better shape?"

A question such as this sends the brain searching for a solution.

Besides what we do consciously, aren't there a lot of times when we're running on automatic pilot? Something is directing us, but we're not sure what it is. The programming in this mode is done by the questions we pose in our own minds.

These aren't the kinds of questions that get big, obvious, immediate answers. This is an undercurrent, a stream of thought that's always flowing though it comes to the surface—to the attention of our conscious mind—only occasionally.

Fill this stream with questions that deliver results you want. "What can I do today, and continue every day, to make a fitness lifestyle a part of my personality?"

You didn't think it was this simple, did you? Don't mistake the simplicity for something easy. A lifetime of thought process can be changed instantly—but it also can revert back just as swiftly. Like a musical instrument, it must be kept in tune. This means steady, consistent action to form the habit of empowering internal queries.

Better questions alone won't get you ready for the Olympics, but they are the key to unlocking the first door that keeps you from attaining a superior fitness level.

Program your mind to set off an alarm when you hear a negative, self-defeating question—and replace it with one that will trigger a solution.

What are you going to do to make your own fitness solution?

There's No Quick Cellulite Solution

Cellulite is the most dreaded word in many a woman's vocabulary. Scientifically, however, cellulite doesn't exist.

Tell that to the legion of women spending millions of dollars on creams, wraps, gloves, exercises, and massages guaranteed to smooth away those dimpled formations on their backsides, and many will brand you a liar.

Up-to-date medical research shows cellulite is simply fat.

Many women have thick layers of fat directly under the skin on their upper thighs and buttocks. And, yes, these thick layers of fat often become dimpled and are difficult to remove. There are scientific ways to attack these problems, but none are quick, easy, or highly advertised.

Cellulite, pronounced *cell*-u-leet, was introduced in the United States by Nicole Ronsard, who in 1973 wrote *Cellulite: Those Lumps, Bumps and Bulges You Couldn't Lose Before.*

Ronsard says cellulite is not regular fat. "It is a gel-like substance made up of fat, water, and wastes trapped in bumpy, immovable pockets just beneath the skin."

I've been over Ronsard's book several times. A page-by-page examination reveals there is little information in the book that appears to be based on scientific fact.

The truth about cellulite:

♦ Cellulite is nothing more than stored fat.

♦ All stored fat, regardless of its location, is hard to remove from the human body.

♦ Women store twice as much fat on their hips and thighs as men do. Much of this is related to hormones and the ability to conceive children.

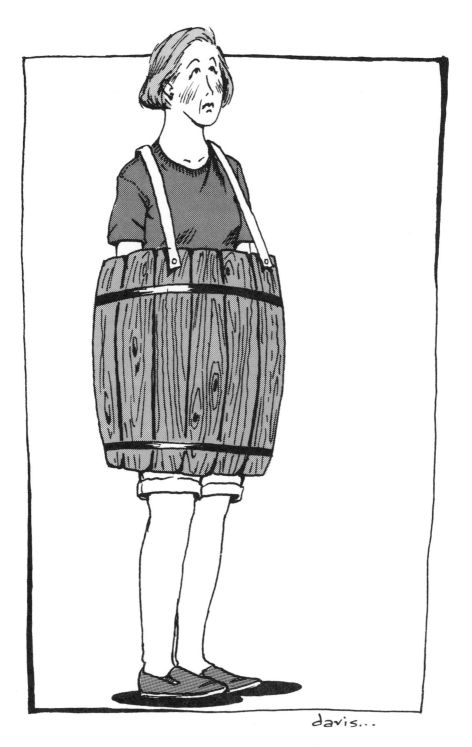

Cellulite is no barrel of fun!

♦ The dimpling effect of the fat on the overlying skin is caused by a combination of over-fatness, loss of muscular size and strength, and the natural aging of connective tissue.

♦ Fat cannot be massaged, perspired, relaxed, soaked, flushed, compressed, or dissolved out of the human body.

Quick and easy solutions to removing dimpled fatty deposits are based on half-truths, myths, ignorance, and outright lies. They do not produce lasting results.

The treatment for dimpled fatty deposits is a two-fold approach:

♦ You must reduce the size of the fat cells by dieting. A well-balanced, descending diet (from 1400 to 1000 calories a day) is the recommended way to reduce.

♦ You must increase the size and strength of the large muscles that compose the hips and thighs. (The other major muscles should also be exercised to support fatty deposits throughout the body.) The most efficient form of exercise is strength training.

85

Small Changes Produce Large Rewards

As kids go back to school, most lives return to normal. The free-and-easy summer schedule slams rudely into the morning alarm clock, and a tightly structured routine takes control of our lives.

This return to discipline may apply to eating and exercising habits, too. If you spent the summer in Margaritaville, your fall wardrobe is probably uncomfortable. Before you're revved into action by disgust, contemplate the powerful effects of small, consistent habit changes.

Think of what it's like to accrue compound interest on an investment. It doesn't seem like much for a while, but the nest egg grows handsomely over time.

Examine your eating pattern. A friend of mine at a party made a valid point a couple of weeks ago, although his remark was received as being facetious. He said he loves German chocolate blizzards from Dairy Queen. He told how he'd get into his car and drive to the Dairy Queen just to get a large German chocolate blizzard, but now that he was on a diet he got a small one.

The listeners at the party chuckled, but we'd all do well to incorporate such a small change into our eating behavior. Austerity is short-lived. Modify only to an extent to which you can adhere long-term.

If you think you can harshly crack down on yourself until you reach your desired weight and then shift into something reasonable, you're reducing your chance of long-term success. The instant-gratification mentality is likely to drive you through cycles of gaining and losing and ending up on a higher plateau of fatness.

Take the steam out of disgust you might feel now and invest it into a marathon of fitness habits instead of a sprint. Check the library or the college bookstores for a nutrition textbook. Several universities publish health/nutrition newsletters or even books.

Shopping the bookstores can be hazardous due to the proliferation of diet fads, but you might find something along the lines of the *Mayo Clinic Family Health Book* or one of the books by Dr. Gabe Mirkin.

Invest the steam of disgust into knowledge.

As for exercise information, see my time-efficient programs which you will find at the bookstores. These programs provide the greatest impact per minute of time invested. The point is, don't go out and run ten miles every morning this next week and eat lettuce and grapefruit. You'll hate exercise, you'll feel miserable, and as soon as you've lost some weight, you'll return to the habits that made you fat and out of shape in the first place.

You'll be in the vicious cycle.

Invest the steam of disgust into bite-size changes to which you can adhere and improve upon methodically over the course of your life.

86

The 10 Percent Change

Habits are a good thing. They cut down on time we would otherwise spend in contemplation, expediting the simple chores.

How quickly would we get ready for work in the morning if we had to think: Do I go into the shower, or do I make coffee? Do I get the newspaper, or do I shut off the alarm?

The routine flows. Driving to work, or taking the kids to school, our conscious mind is on the day's activities while our subconscious is at the controls of the automobile. Auto piloting is shifted immediately from sub-conscious to conscious, however, when someone pulls out in front of us at an intersection.

We are, indeed, creatures of habits. Good habits and bad habits, alike. The habits that produce a sedentary lifestyle and permit an "over fat" body are worth changing. But just like our morning wake-up routine, these are rutted in deep grooves that are not easily replanted.

To overcome the frustration prevalent in a habit-changing endeavor, envision the results of just a 10 percent habit improvement. Not a tempo-rary 10 percent habit improvement, but a permanent one. The change is so subtle that there's less frustration in the initial attempt. This provides a good shot at long-term success.

Making a 10-percent change today may not seem like much, but will make a big difference in where you are five years from now. A 10-percent change compounds itself like interest on money. Make this your body's IRA.

What constitutes a 10-percent improvement in your eating habits? Maybe it's a reduction in saturated fat intake from whole milk to skim, from ice cream to frozen yogurt, from beef to fowl.

Maybe it's a stronger commitment or a commitment to a regular exer-cise program.

Ten percent is whatever you judge to be of minor significance, but significant nonetheless.

Identify areas of possible habit improvement by making a list. "Some of my less-than-ideal eating/exercising habits are _____"

What do these habits keep you from doing or achieving? How do they make you feel? Record a statement to yourself.

What are you willing to do to make a permanent change? You may slip from time to time, but when you do, collect yourself and return to your plan of action.

Make sure the change you target is only 10 percent. Trying to be per-fect will frustrate you into greater imperfection.

A 10-percent change makes a graduated improvement that com-pounds itself. A daily net caloric deficit of just 100 calories per day (a table-spoon of mayonnaise) reduces ten pounds of body fat in a year.

If you want to be ten pounds thinner by this time next year—and stay that way—stop trying to be twenty pounds thinner by next month.

It requires some effort to make this habit change initially, but once in place it will flow smoothly.

Our habits can be good, bad, or indifferent. We're always going to have a supply in each category. The goal is to shift a manageable amount of the BAD column off the ledger.

Put your body's IRA, your 10-percent habit-improvement plan, into action right away. You'll start reaping the benefit even before retirement.

Don't Let Winter Get Under Your Skin

Winter can be detrimental to your skin. Wind, cold, and dry heated indoor air strip your skin of moisture, leaving it vulnerable to chapping, redness, and flaking. Exercising outdoors in winter weather makes skin care even trickier because sweat, wind, and sun can dry and burn the skin.

To keep your skin supple and nourished, daily care is a must. Here are some helpful guidelines:

♦ Drink at least a gallon of water each day. I've mentioned this previously as an important aspect of fat loss. It's equally important in nourishing your skin.

A sixteen-ounce plastic bottle with a straw facilitates your water drinking. Most people find they can consume more fluid with a straw than they can by drinking from a glass. A great way to keep up with your water drinking is to place rubber bands around the middle of the bottle equal to the number of bottles of water you are supposed to drink. Each time you finish sixteen ounces, take off a rubber band.

♦ Apply a moisturizer morning and night and before and after exercising. There are a myriad of products available. Exotic ingredients like elastin, collagen, mink oil, DNA, and unpronounceable formulas increase the cost of the product but not its effectiveness. Research proves that nothing is better at moisturizing the skin than simple cold cream or petroleum jelly. Be sure and check the label for desired ingredients.

♦ Use a sunblock when working or exercising outdoors.

♦ Avoid long, hot showers. They wash protective fluids from your skin. A warm bath is much better. Use a moisturizing cleaner to better absorb and hold your skin's fluids.

♦ Understand that no lotion, creme, or moisturizer will work quickly on the toughened skin that you may have on your elbows and feet. Such toughened areas can be treated through bodybraising, which removes built-up layers of dead skin. For best results, see a skin-care professional.

Be good to your skin from head to toe. Water it, cleanse it, moisturize it, and protect it.

Your reward will be self-evident.

88

Get Extra Pounds to Take a Hike

I've never been much of a believer in walking as an effective method of exercise.

Walking does nothing for your strength or flexibility. It can produce a benefit to your cardiovascular endurance, but only if you walk uphill at a fast pace. Even then, there are certain uphill-downhill dangers and impact forces that may offset the benefit.

Nor is walking an efficient way to burn calories. At least I didn't believe it was until I applied the results of a study by Dr. J. Mark Davis and colleagues from the Department of Exercise Sciences, University of South Carolina.

Dr. Davis measured and compared the energy expenditure for three hours of seven women after the following treatments: exercise only, meal only, exercise-meal, and meal-exercise. The results showed that the meal-exercise routine increased energy expenditure among the women by an average of 30 percent, compared to the other treatments.

The researchers concluded that going for a walk after you eat brings on exercise-induced "post-prandial thermogenesis," which means the production of extra body heat produced by exercising on a full stomach.

After studying this thermogenic effect with 100 women involved in my *Two Weeks to a Tighter Tummy* research program, some surprising findings emerged. Most women I've worked with in the past are elated if they can lose two pounds of fat a week on a combination diet and exercise program. With my new plan, which included walking, the average fat loss was 3.51

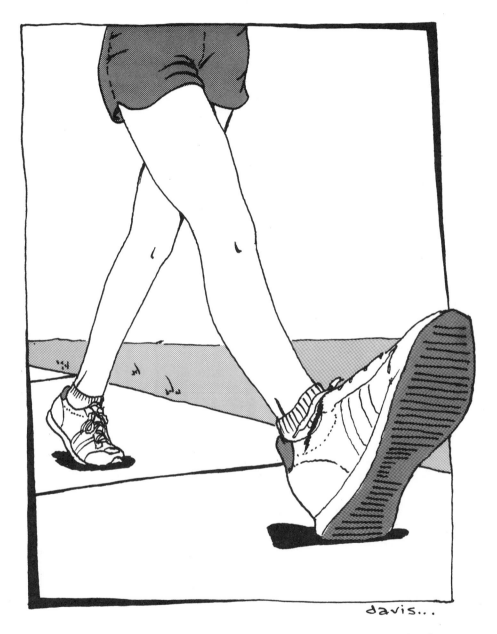

Walking after your evening meal can speed up your body's fat-burning mechanism.

pounds per week. That's a 75 percent improvement in fat loss, and the losses were typical throughout the 100 women. At the extreme, seven of the ten women lost more than five pounds of fat per week—or 10 pounds in two weeks!

To speed up the calorie-burning mechanism, here's what to do:

♦ Eat your normal evening meal.

♦ Begin your walk within fifteen minutes after you finish your meal.

♦ Walk at a leisurely pace for only thirty minutes. How far should you walk at such a pace? A leisurely pace would cover from 1½ to 2 miles.

♦ Carry an insulated water bottle with you and drink at least 16 ounces of cold water as you walk.

♦ Wear well-constructed, well-cushioned, comfortable walking or running shoes. Do not wear street shoes.

♦ Dress in lightweight, comfortable clothes.

♦ Walk outdoors, if possible, on level ground. Or you may substitute a bicycle ride for a walk. If the weather is a problem, you may walk indoors, or use a stationary bicycle or treadmill.

Try the eating-walking-watering routine each day for two weeks and you'll be hooked on thermogensis.

In a real sense you'll be walking fat away!

Fighting Fat Hips and Thighs Takes All-around Effort

Why can't you seem to lose the fat around your (choose one):

♦ Thighs

♦ Waist

♦ Hips

♦ Back of upper arms

♦ Breasts

Though most other areas of your body seem to be relatively fat-free, pouches of flab still remain in an area you've come to consider your trouble spot. And it bothers you.

Fat stored in the body can be made from any food component (carbohydrates, fats, or proteins). When food is eaten, it travels to the stomach and intestines. Enzymes break down the food into glucose, amino acids and minute droplets of fat. The fats then travel to the liver, where they are processed.

From the liver, the fats enter the circulatory system, where they can be used for energy by many organs.

Excess fats will be stored in adipose cells. When more energy is needed, fats are released, according to the fat-ordering process programmed into your genes. If the need continues, the cells will shrink but they remain.

But why can't you shed the fat from a particular area? One theory is that each fat cell in your body has two kinds of receptors on its surface. Alpha receptors stimulate fat accumulation, while the beta receptors stimulate fat breakdown. But those receptors are not equal; one dominates the other.

Your trouble spot probably contains fat cells dominated by alpha receptors, which means they excel in accumulating fat. And they are very reluctant—stubborn, in fact—to mobilize fat for energy. The best strategy is to build your muscle mass in your skinny area to fill it out, combined with reducing calorie intake to burn fat from the stubborn area.

You may, however, have to live with being too fat in one area or too skinny in another. It depends on the severity of your fat distribution disparity.

And what about the spot-reducing exercises promoted on TV and in the tabloids at the grocery checkout? You know, sit-ups for a protruding belly, side bends for the love handles, and leg lifts for those thunder thighs?

Despite these insinuations, the scientific literature has never been ambivalent about this; there is no such thing as spot reduction. Feeling muscle burn in a particular area does not mean the nearby fat has been incinerated. Your liver determines which fat cells are mobilized. And it has a pecking order all its own, programmed into your genes.

Studies with people doing hundreds of sit-ups, and on comparing tennis players' racket arms to a non-racket arms, have shown that you cannot pinpoint the shrinkage of adipose tissue.

But don't give up on exercise. Strengthen all your muscles, particularly the large muscle groups. Every pound of muscle you add will burn an additional 75 calories a day, even at rest. If you manage your eating to create a net calorie deficit, you will burn body fat. With a gradual, lower-calorie diet combined with proper strength training, your trouble sports will be conquered.

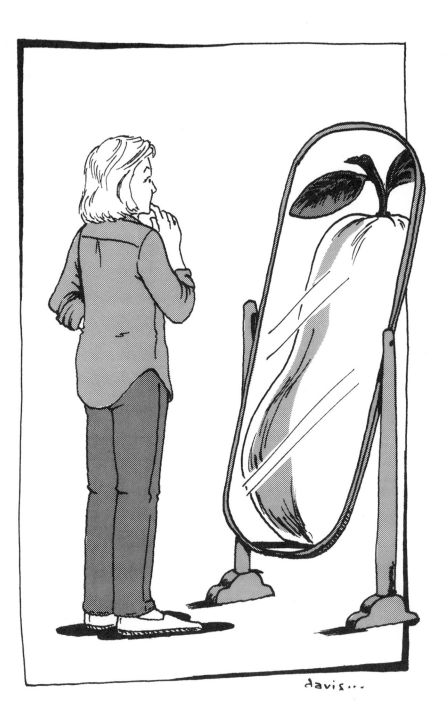

What is your basic body type?

90

Paring Down Apple and Pear Shapes

If your figure doesn't make you a candidate for a magazine swimsuit issue, is it because you're shaped like an apple or a pear? Fat above and around the waist signifies the contour of an apple. Pear shape means a mass of hip, thigh, and buttock bulges.

The location of your fat concentration has a definite meaning.

Apples are luckier than pears in that they stand a better chance of reducing their fat. However, fat accumulation in the abdominal cavity is an indication of increased health risks.

Conversely, pears do not have the health hazards of those with fat bellies, but they have a tougher time reducing the size of their hips and thighs.

Women dominate the pear-shaped physiques, while men are more likely to be apples. But the issue does not split precisely among the gender line; women can be apples and men can be pears.

Hip, thigh, and buttock fat is usually subcutaneous, which means it is stored directly beneath the skin. It is very soft to touch.

Apples store their fat within the abdominal cavity, pushing the abdominal muscles outward. This is why big bellies often feel hard, like a basketball.

Once the abdominal cavity is filled, apples start storing subcutaneous fat in other areas.

There is a popular myth about a fat belly pulling on your heart, creating a coronary risk. A fat belly is indeed a coronary risk, but not because it is going to yank your heart out of place.

Enzyme action moves fat easily in and out of fat cells in the abdominal cavity. During exercise, this fat is directed toward the working muscles, via the bloodstream. During times of emotional stress, however, fat-laden blood from the abdominal cavity goes to the liver, providing it with abundant raw material for the production of cholesterol.

Further bad news for apples is that fat cells in the abdominal region tend to be larger than those in other areas of the body. Large fat cells are associated with glucose intolerance and an excess of insulin in the blood, which can develop into diabetes.

Excess insulin may cause the kidneys to reabsorb sodium, which may lead to high blood pressure.

Apples face a greater risk of heart attack than do pears. But the good news for apples is that they have an easier time getting rid of their fat.

A 1988 study showed that male apples could reduce body fat through exercise without caloric restriction. Women, especially those who are pear-shaped, have to restrict calorie intake along with exercise.

One study, in fact, showed that fat cells in the female gluteal-femoral pattern are very stubborn, except during lactation. This suggests that the female body guards its fat cells to ensure adequate energy support for a nursing baby.

As a means of assessing your health risk, measure your waist and your hips.

Consider your waist to be the narrowest part on your torso. Your hip measurement should be the largest circumference around your hips and buttocks.

Now, divide your waist measurement by your hip measurement. Hopefully, your waist is smaller than your hips. This means your resulting number is less than one, a point something or other.

If your waist is twenty-four inches and your hips are thirty-six, the ratio is .66. From a health-risk standpoint, this is good. But if your waist measurement is thirty-nine inches, and your hips thirty-four, the red lights and sirens should start wailing—your waist-to-hip ratio is 1.15. Time to start exercising!

91

Males' Genes Affect Longevity

Why are there more boy babies than girl babies, but more elderly women than elderly men? This is a question that concerns not only lonely widows but also one insightful anthropologist.

In his book, *The Natural Superiority of Women,* Ashley Montagu listed more than thirty serious disorders in males caused by abnormalities in sex-linked genes, ranging from nearsightedness to heart defects.

"To commence life as a male," wrote Montagu, "is to start off with a disadvantage—a disadvantage that operates at every stage of life."

Even without awareness of Montagu's work, most men I know would readily agree. But there are reasons they've never realized.

The greater male mortality begins even before birth. It's estimated that 30 percent more male embryos are conceived than females. As many as 75 percent of all embryos die before the mother realizes she is pregnant.

One theory is that immunological differences between mother and son are greater than those between mother and daughter, resulting in a greater number of male embryos being rejected by the mother's body.

Still, 105 males are born to every 100 females. But in every age group beginning in infancy, the death rate for males is higher than that for females.

By age 35 females outnumber males, and the gap widens as the years progress. By age 75, three women are alive for every two men.

A female born in 1950 had a life expectancy of 71 years; a male born the same year could expect 5.5 fewer birthdays. Babies of 1986 vintage show a seven-year female advantage, 78.5 years to 71.5.

Males tend to eat more, drink more, smoke more, and undergo more stress, some researchers point out. But besides these lifestyle factors, women have a biological advantage.

The X chromosome (the female sex chromosome) carries other important genes that the Y chromosome (male) does not. Hence, males suffer disproportions from genetic errors, which can raise the risk of fatal illness throughout life.

The male sex hormone, testosterone, also works against longevity. It is testosterone that causes the male to excite more easily than the female, to be aggressive and competitive, and to engage in risky behavior. In the late teens and early twenties, male death rates are three times those of females, mostly due to violent deaths such as suicide, homicide, and automobile accidents.

Estelle Ramey, a physiologist who worked for many years at Georgetown University, says that heightened response puts more wear and tear on the male body, particularly the cardiovascular system. "Every time it happens," Ramey said, "men do a little bit of damage to the lining of their blood vessels. That damage begins to accumulate. It's the price men pay for their ability to react quickly to a threat."

Estrogen, says Ramey, gives women a fifteen-year advantage in terms of cardiovascular disease.

The biological disadvantages should encourage men to be more diligent in their lifestyle habits. Prudent eating and productive exercise may make a difference.

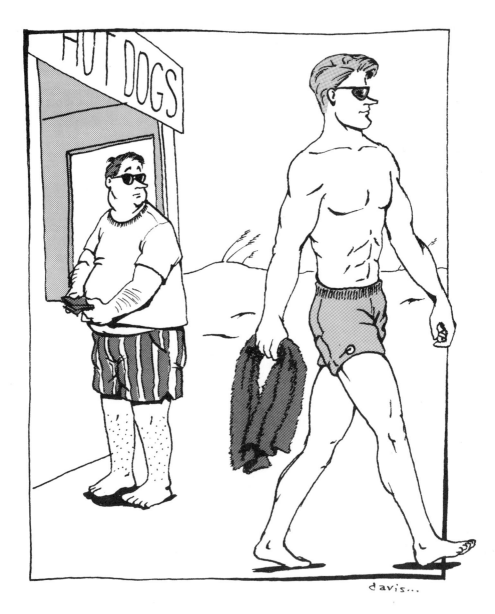

"Hmmmm . . . on second thought, you can hold the chili."

92

The Way to a Trim Waist

Synergism is the simultaneous occurrence of separate factors that together have greater effect than the sum of their individual actions.

Synergism is a major reason for the dramatic body composition changes in 146 men from Dallas who participated in my 32-day fat-loss, muscle-building program.

The men followed an eating plan providing 1500 to 1400 calories per day and exercised at a high level of intensity under one-on-one supervision on a circuit of Nautilus machines three times per week.

The average man in this group was forty years old and weighed almost 200 pounds at the start. In thirty-two days, he dropped 17.07 pounds of fat, trimmed 3.03 inches off the waist and packed on 3.65 pounds of muscle.

Inspiring pictures of these men, before and after, are presented in my book, *32 Days to a 32-Inch Waist* (Taylor Publishing, $8.95).

They are testimony to what can be done when you really want to lose fat and when you have someone pushing you to a maximum effort each workout.

The effects of the 32/32 reduction plan combined with the 32/32 exercises are excellent examples of synergism. Simultaneously losing fat and building muscle produces at least three important results: guaranteed fat loss, increased metabolic rate, and improved body shape.

Like a basketball team, the blend is very potent.

There's a disclaimer that accompanies the book's title. Achieving a 32-inch waist in thirty-two days is realistic only if you're within 4 or 5 inches of 32 inches. One man lost 6 inches in thirty-two days, from 45 inches to 39. Another man went through three consecutive rounds of the program, trimming almost 11 inches off his waist while shedding more than 36 pounds of fat.

So, what are your fitness goals this month? Might this be a worthwhile project to try?

The idea of a 32-inch waist is based on it being the girth measurement most men were graced with in high school. Like a beacon calling you home, this book provides the step-by-step instructions for turning back the years, or at least the inches.

93

When Fat and Forty Set In

The most profound birthday for taking stock of our physical well being seems to be the big 4–0, especially for women. This crisis usually includes the realization that your twenty-year-old figure is definitely two decades behind you.

If 4–0 is fast approaching, here is a scenario that might sound familiar.

Mary is a thirty-eight-year-old mother who works full-time as a nurse in addition to her domestic duties. Excepting her two pregnancies, Mary has remained a size 10 since her early twenties. Within the past year, however, her hips, thighs, and tummy have blossomed, or so it seems to Mary.

Although she applied dietary restrictions that worked in the past, Mary eventually had to concede her new dimensions and purchase size twelve pants.

Having maintained a size 10 for so many years, Mary was sure one size larger would never become too small. But within another six months, Mary was bursting at the seams of her size 12s. She now had to shift up to—ugh—a size 14.

Panic overwhelmed Mary. Calories became her enemy. She ate as few as she possibly could, starving herself on and off cycles for a period of eighteen months. Her scale reinforced this behavior by registering lower numbers. Mary gravitated to diet programs that promised quick weight loss.

The fictitious Mary represents the typical mind-set of the average American woman. Her problem is compounded by her failure to realize that this is not a sudden crisis. Mary's fatness is actually an insidious dilemma, originating many years earlier.

Unless Mary had performed a regimen of quality strength training in her adult years, her muscle-to-fat ratio was its highest between the ages of sixteen to twenty. During this time she had approximately 2.5 pounds of muscle for each pound of fat. This 2.5/1 ratio is due to hormones, nutrition, and vigorous daily activities.

As Mary aged her muscles deteriorated primarily from a slowdown of activity. Meanwhile, her body fat increased because of this loss of calorie-burning muscle as well as the reduced activity and probably a little more of "the good life." However, Mary felt secure about her figure for many years, because her scale weight remained at a magic number: perhaps 125 pounds.

But Mary's figure had been steadily reproportioning itself. Her hips, once held high and firm with muscle, slowly fell into a shapeless, baggy bottom. Simultaneously, Mary collected a paunch of fat just below the navel.

The space in Mary's slacks that was once filled by her shapely hips in the rear was now occupied by the paunch of fat in the front.

So slowly had Mary's figure been changing, however, that she had not detected the shifting sands of time. Little by little she had been fitting differently into the size she had always worn. In fact, her clothes tended to support and hide her worsening proportions.

Once Mary arrived at the edge of her size 10s, increasing sizes began to happen much more rapidly. But it was self-deceiving for her to think that she had suddenly outgrown her wardrobe. By resorting to crash dieting, Mary achieved short-term scale weight losses by suffered long-term metabolism damage. Yo-yo dieting was under way.

Mary's damaged metabolism accelerated her storage of fat, causing her to increase several more sizes before reaching age forty. When she assesses her physical well being, it won't be an uplifting experience.

Next, we'll examine five mistakes in Mary's thinking, and what she can do to correct them.

94

Fitness Outweighs Dieting At Forty

Last chapter we were discussing the scenario of a woman approaching her fortieth birthday with a sense of panic as her clothing size seemed to increase rapidly.

But the increase was very slow, not rapid. Mary's figure had been reproportioning itself for many years. She had been losing muscle and gaining fat, shifting around in her size-10 pants. Then the dam burst and Mary started increasing sizes at an alarming rate.

Mary's affliction is shared by most women. It is a natural maturation and aging effect, exacerbated by ignorance, social practice, and myth.

Mary must understand the following:

♦ Fatness is often not a matter of steady gorging. Like most overly fat people, Mary had said to herself incredulously, "but I don't eat that much!" Excess fat usually results from overeating a little bit for a long time, coupled with a lifestyle that made no effort to at least maintain muscle mass.

    The average woman between the ages of twenty and forty loses ten pounds of muscle, or one-half pound per year. If her body weight remains the same, she gains ten pounds of fat over the same twenty years.

♦ The bathroom scale told Mary only one thing—her body weight. It did not tell her how much of her weight was fat compared to bone, vital organs, and muscle. A pound of muscle fits tightly against the body, adding shape and firmness. A pound of fat just sort of hangs in a glob taking up 20 percent more space than one pound of muscle. But the scale weighs each as one pound.

    Emphasis must be placed on body composition—the ratio of muscle to fat—and not weight.

♦ "Weight" loss programs are meaningless. The issue is fat, not weight. A woman weighing 150 pounds wearing a size 9/10 is much different from a woman weighing 150 pounds wearing a size 15/16. The difference is in body-shaping muscle, which can be achieved only through an effective strength-training program.

♦ Crash dieting worsens the problem. Each time Mary starved herself her body cannibalized muscle mass for energy, almost as much as it mobilized fat stores. Each pound of cannibalized muscle lowered Mary's basal metabolism by 75 calories per day. Her body's prehistoric time clock also shifted into starvation mode, further lowering metabolism.

♦ Mary probably misunderstood the role of exercise, believing that its purpose is to burn calories. Mary would have to run for thirty-five to fifty miles to burn a single pound of fat. The first purpose of exercise is to force the body to increase, or at least maintain, its calorie-burning muscle mass. When calorie consumption is below its daily expenditure, the body will just as likely burn muscle as fat for energy, unless there is a demand placed on the muscles to increase in size and strength.

The solution to the Fat-and-Forty Syndrome is simple but not easy. Mary needs to strengthen her muscles while eating a moderate-calorie, well-balanced diet. She should keep track of inches and firmness along with total body weight.

She cannot allow herself to be victimized by the lure of "quick-and-easy" solutions. If quick-and-easy solutions exist, why are there overfat people?

Mary needs to make a lifestyle change. She must prudently manage her calorie intake and make regular strengthening exercises as second nature as her various hygiene habits.

But there is hope. If Mary is sensible, reasonable, and patient, she may just rediscover her twenty-year-old figure. Instead of fat and forty, she'll become firm and fit.

Quality Concerns for The Gift of Fitness

If you're considering slipping a fitness-related gift under the tree, *caveat emptor* (let the buyer beware).

Do you have input and direction from the recipient? Exercise and eating disciplines are very personal habits. You can avoid recipient's remorse if you have clear indications on what they want and are willing to use.

Would the gift make a difference? Is he/she committed to a fitness routine of any sort right now? If they are, your gift could enhance their efforts, but if they haven't mastered any fitness habit, it's likely the gift will be a short-lived novelty.

Fitness equipment in the home tends to become a monument to good intention. Just look at classified ads of people selling exercise bikes and rowers. There are too many other things to do at home, and too many distractions are possible even if you do commence exercising.

When you were in college, did you notice that your best studying was done at the library, or some other quiet place away from home? We are creatures of associations. We have to associate a time and a place for exercise, and the many purposes of our homes do not lend themselves to the conquering of a single-minded purpose.

The alternative is a health club membership or professional instruction. But the purpose of this article is to navigate you through catalogue and store merchandise that often looks great and functions poorly.

If I haven't dissuaded you from buying a piece of equipment, don't be suckered by pretty pictures. Merchandisers always show their product being used by some phenomenal physique, and we believe the advertised device is responsible. If you think the amazing something or other for $19.95 will give you the body of the person in the commercial, I have some bonds that will enable you to retire in three months.

Beware of component parts in exercise equipment. Multi-station exercise machines, especially, are just pretty pieces of junk if their joints are comprised merely of bolts passing through metal. They should at least have bushings, if not bearings, in all pivotal points. This criterion generally wipes out all devices priced at less than a thousand dollars.

The most economical muscle-building means, incidentally is a set of barbells and a stable bench. But make sure the person knows how to use free weights properly. Many teen-age boys, especially develop lifetime nagging injuries from misusing or abusing weight-training equipment.

The best-selling home devices the last several years, however, target cardiovascular training, not strength development.

Plan to spend several hundred dollars if you want a quality bike. Cheaper ones usually vibrate or are loaded with an intolerable level of friction. They also tend to have seats without springs underneath, and derriere endurement will be a problem. These product deficiencies can be deceiving. You'll quit using the bike without being able to pinpoint your dissatisfaction, mistakenly blaming it on a lack of discipline.

Instead of an upright bike, test-ride one that is recumbent, that is, one in which the exerciser sits reclined. Holding your legs out in front of you while pedalling requires greater muscle action (especially from the hips) than do legs that dangle from an upright seat. This means you'll use greater energy (calories) per revolution.

Home steppers, stair climbers, and ski simulators also need to be scrutinized for quality. Without being a mechanical engineer, the bottom line on the issue is money-back guarantee and warranty. Be sure to weigh these factors into your decision.

It's easy to get suckered into low-grade exercise equipment. The untrained eye and budget mind are poor decipherers of quality.

A set of pushup handles for about a dozen dollars, a book with illustrated floor exercises, and a swanky exercise outfit might settle the confusion, don't you think?

Then again, there's always socks and underwear.

96

A Slim Body Can Make a Difference in Business

From the standpoint of job performance, have you ever stopped to calculate the high cost of being overfat?

We've heard many times that abundant adipose tissue sucks vitality right out of our cellular structure. But the good times can roll for years before our health dwindles prematurely. So we'll worry later.

Meanwhile, there is a more immediate reason we might want to slice off a few inches.

Excess body fat sends signals that hamper our relationships with other people. First impressions might not be everything, but a poor one sure takes a long time to overcome. No matter how smart, sincere, or wonderful we are, our appearance acts as a filter through which everything else is judged.

Dressing for success means our clothing had better be of moderate size, as well as the right color, style, and fabric.

Women who wouldn't be caught dead with a mismatch of shoes and handbag nonetheless waddle around town going about their business. Men sure to wear a silk tie in a power color still feel no shame about draping it over a basketball belly.

There are very few professions in which we're not dealing with people. To a significant degree, we're always trying to influence those around us—even our children—in some way.

Rightfully or wrongfully, a slender physique tells the world that discipline and motivation reside inside. True or not, it matters very little, because the perception might as well be the reality.

Physiology speaks, even before we do. If anything the least bit articulate comes out of the mouth of a slender body, the intelligence is assessed in glowing terms.

The exact same words out of an overfat body don't land with as much impact. The person we're encountering will have skepticism: If this person is so sharp, why don't they do something to lose weight?

We generally want people we're dealing with to have confidence in us, do we not?

Physiology can be an asset, or a liability, or maybe it's just neutral. We don't have to become obsessed with winning a physique or bikini contest. The right business suit is a great equalizer, so long as the body inside is within shooting distance of its ideal muscle-to-fat ratio.

If your boss hasn't told you to lose weight, it's probably because he or she doesn't want to have to shape up, either. If your doctor hasn't told you to lose weight, it's probably because he or she would be embarrassed.

Boldly facing reality is the catharsis we all need. And there's more good news.

The two-pronged process of shedding fat—exercising and eating better—delivers another business bonanza: more energy.

Our slimmer, more energized bodies might be enough to push us through some barriers. Most of us are in a situation where 10 percent greater effort would produce not 10-percent greater results—but 100 percent.

Physiology indeed speaks. Better make sure yours is saying something good about you.

97

Nine Ways to Help You Spring Back into Shape

At picnics, pool parties, the beach, working in the yard, on the boat, and wherever else the sun beats down on us relentlessly, a lot of body will be showing as summer arrives.

But the hibernation of our diligent eating habits has left a 5- to 10-pound residue in places that can no longer be hidden in a winter wardrobe.

In lieu of panic, try this nine-point spring tuneup:

♦ Drink plenty of water, it is the closest thing to a magic fat-loss potion. Sixty-four ounces per day is an absolute minimum; even three times that is desirable. Drink water even when you think you're not thirsty.

♦ Besides water, chew whatever calories you consume, don't drink them. Studies show that we need the oral gratification of chewing. This is why so-called liquid meal replacement offer no sustainable solution.

Water and even black coffee and tea have no calories, and diet soft drinks have either none or just a few. Be careful with the diet drinks, however, because the artificial sweeteners can trigger cravings in some people.

This chew-calorie proviso especially means no alcohol. No matter how conservative you are in your calorie consumption, alcohol will crowd out fat mobilization by consuming your liver's full attention.

♦ Stay out of restaurants where you gorge yourself. Even if you intend to eat sensibly, walking into a dining establishment where you typically enjoy a mega-calorie favorite is setting yourself up for ambush. If you must eat in a restaurant, try one you've never been to before, and call ahead to pick out a sensible selection.

♦ Rearrange your kitchen cabinets. Scramble your behavior patterns by putting snacks in different locations. Then when you're operating on automatic pilot, the cookies won't be there and you'll be jarred into remembering your fat-loss goal.

♦ Don't buy any clothing that comfortably absorbs your new, expanded dimensions. Conversely, try on your tightest-fitting clothes at least once a week.

♦ Pick an exercise you can stick with, but be careful if it's swimming (or anything in water). While swimming offers exercise, the thermal effect of being submerged in water is likely to cause you to eat more.

♦ Don't over exercise. Depending on the intensity, three times per week is plenty, at no more than 20 to 30 minutes each. Too much exercise tears down body tissue, increases injury risk, and will thus make you inactive over the long term.

♦ Get out from in front of the TV. A good book and extended daylight hours will help this. Decreasing our exposure to a billion-dollar advertising industry diminishes the temptations to impulsively overeat.

♦ Take to heart some advice borrowed from author Zig Ziglar:

"Life demands before it rewards. You've got to be before you can do, you've got to do before you can have. When you're tough on yourself, life becomes easy . . . You don't pay the price for good health, you enjoy the benefits of it—you pay the price for poor health."

======================= 98 =======================

Good Habits That Last Come in Stages

Maybe you've struggled so many times in the past that now it seems like a quantum leap from fatness to fitness. Countless times you've fired your engine, cranked your motivation, roared down the runway and fallen flat on your face just a few feet from your point of take-off.

It's like the newsreels we see of the forerunners to the Wright Brothers. Before Orville and Wilbur finally succeeded, they and many others failed.

Author Zig Ziglar would tell us that anything worth doing is worth doing poorly . . . until we get good at it. The same applies to the fitness lifestyle we may desire.

Change is difficult, but change is what's required if we're dissatisfied with our health, energy level or body composition. We have to discipline ourselves and do things that make us uncomfortable for a while.

Research on addictive behaviors shows that there are four stages in changing lifestyle habits. These are:

♦ **Precontemplation**
Motivation and commitment begin to develop in this stage. There is abundant desire, but confidence is low. Dieting requires a full-time commitment, and we must decide whether the other factors in our lives provide a good opportunity to concentrate on modifying lifestyle habits deeply ingrained in our psyches.

♦ **Contemplation**
Confidence and motivation shift into the moderate-to-high range during this stage. We assess our fat attitudes and behaviors. We then perform a step that is critical: We identify and prioritize the habits that requires modification. Failing to do this would be like taking a seat in a cockpit without any controls and instrumentation to navigate our journey.

♦ **Action**
We start at the bottom—not at the top—of our priority list of habits that need changing. Bite off the small steps first, building momentum for the more challenging ones. Goals are clearly defined. Just as with our

finances, keeping records is a must. A journal of everything is the most effective tool of analysis. Through this we can identify our emotional triggers that set off binges. Without it there is no manual to tell us how our machinery operates.

♦ **Maintenance**

Our confidence and motivation levels fluctuate widely, but we've basically adopted healthier habits. The danger is that we prematurely conclude that we've mastered the skills of lifelong fitness management. The winds will change, and there will be new storms to encounter. The learning never ends.

Now is the time to perfect the art of lapsing without relapsing. A lapse is a brief interlude of overindulgence from which there is a quick and decisive recovery. Relapse occurs when lapses string together such that it's the rule instead of an exception. When relapse is complete, collapse occurs and the old fat behavior returns in full force.

Recognizing the four stages of change should help us build a solid foundation before embarking on one of life's most challenging journeys.

After all, Orville and Wilbur did not take flight without a great many trials and errors. If you've done a poor job of changing habits many times in the past, let the experience be a teacher instead of a reason for discouragement.

Soon you'll not only be flying, you'll be soaring!

Overlearning
Is the Key

Soft steps, small steps, easy-to-understand steps.
    You've examined the many steps that compose this book. Now it's up to you to apply them to your lifestyle. It's time for you to take control.

The best way to take control is by overlearning.

Overlearning simply means the practicing of the steps, guidelines, or skills again and again until they're so ingrained that almost nothing can disturb them.

Giving up a high-calorie snack for one day is a successful small step, as is the second and third day's abstinence. Other examples are being consistent in your strength-training workouts, drinking your water each day, walking after your evening meal, and many others—all of which relate to small, but visible, success. By adding enough of these small steps together, you can build a strong shield against temptations to return to your old ways of coping.

Understand, apply, practice, and **overlearn!**

Each day your soft steps can move you closer and closer to a hard body. A hard body is most definitely in your future.

Once you get that hard body you've always desired, these same soft steps will allow you to keep your body hard permanently. Overlearning your soft steps allows you to persist even when stressful life events emerge to the forefront.

Your body matters. Your fitness matters. Your health matters.

Overlearning is the key.

No one cares about you and your body as much as you do.

Take control now!

ABOUT THE AUTHOR

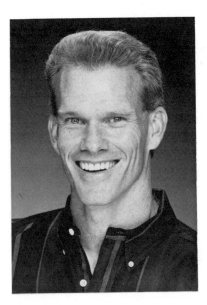

He is the Renaissance man of fitness: an athlete with brains, a disciplinarian with heart, and a scientist with regard for both mind and body. He is Ellington Darden, Ph.D., founding Director of Research for Nautilus Sports/ Medical Industries, author of thirty-eight books on physical fitness, and leading expert on strength training.

Through his programs and courses, he transforms the weak and the willing into the strong and the robust. It isn't easy, but with Dr. Darden's unwavering support and a little bit of self-discipline, participants can metamorphosize their bodies into better shape than they'd ever imagined. This, in turn, escalates them many steps down the road to life-long health and vitality.

Dr. Darden's outstanding research was recognized in 1989 when he was honored as one of the top ten health leaders in the United States by the President's Council on Physical Fitness and Sports.

He received his bachelor's and master's degrees in physical education from Baylor University. He studied five years at Florida State University, where he earned his doctorate in exercise science and completed two years of post-doctorate work in food and nutrition.

As a man tirelessly dedicated to improving the physical well-being of his clients, Dr. Darden reveals only one regret.

"I wish I could change more lives, and change them faster. There's such an overabundance of misunderstanding out there, and it just seems to get bigger every day. Sometimes I feel I need to stand in the middle of the freeway, stop every car, and tell people how important it is to take care of their bodies. Somehow, someway, I've got to make my voice heard above all the riffraff. It is my personal challenge to accomplish this in my lifetime."

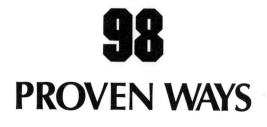

98

PROVEN WAYS

TO TAKE CONTROL
OF YOUR

BODY FITNESS!